Numb Toes and Other Woes

Numb Toes and Other Woes:

More On Peripheral Neuropathy

(Volume 2 in the Numb Toes Series)

By
John A. Senneff

MedPress
Halifax, Nova Scotia

Published by
MedPress
www.medpress.com

Library of Congress Control Number: 2001116939

ISBN (pbk.): 0-9781820-2-2
ISBN (hrdbk.): 0-9781820-3-0

This text is printed on acid-free paper.

Printed in the United States of America.

10 9 8 7 6 5 4 3 2

To my sweet wife, Beth, who helped in countless ways in bringing both this book and Numb Toes and Aching Soles, to completion.

Contents

Foreword to Foreword

I feel fortunate in having Dr. Richard Marks write the foreword to this book. Being both a victim of peripheral neuropathy himself and a physician, he brings a dual perspective to the subject of PN. However, it is the particular area of practice in which he was engaged for 45 years with such distinction—oncology—that makes his insights so relevant. As a cancer specialist he dealt with chronic pain daily; dealing with chronic pain is a prime focus of this book.

Dr. Marks had an illustrious career in oncology before his own pain and related problems caused by peripheral neuropathy became so debilitating that he was forced to retire. He was the medical director of the Columbia Trident Cancer Center, Charleston, South Carolina; chairman and professor of radiation therapy, Medical University of South Carolina; medical director and president of the board, Hospice of Charleston; state president, South Carolina Division of the American Cancer Society; and very active in his own medical practice. And that is just a partial listing of his many medical and volunteer activities.

It's nice to have such a highly regarded expert on your side. But to tell you the truth, the reason I feel so fortunate in having Dr. Marks write for this book was his willingness to share his very personal experiences in a warm and human way. He clearly understands what giving of your self can do for others. As he writes in his foreword, “People with grief, hopelessness, and despair, need love, a little light in the tunnel, a hug, and some proper pain relief.” That kind of says it all.

John Senneff

Foreword

Before I comment on this book, *Numb Toes and Other Woes,* I must comment on the author. From a former oncology department chairman, director of a residency program, medical director of a Hospice, and a practicing physician for 45 years, I am humbled and awed by the information displayed here. I have never met John Senneff, but I know his age and he is wise beyond his years. Despite his disease for eighteen years, the effort and energy to compile all of this information about pain and the control of pain, is unbelievable. *Numb Toes and Aching Soles,* his first book, has been my Bible. This new book will become my textbook and should be for every patient, caregiver or teacher of peripheral neuropathy. He covers the problem of pain with candor, authority, and humor. The following story will reveal why I have had the privilege of reading this book and making my comments.

I knew something was seriously wrong with me, but I was ignorant and in denial. Doctors, friends, and family said it was depression. Depression can be produced by disappointments in life, but they usually go away and depression due to chemical imbalances is treated by new improved drugs. There is a huge difference between depression and grief, hopelessness, and despair. The latter caused me to tell my wife about ten months ago that I was considering suicide. Her response was one you would expect, with shock and alarm, she told me to see a psychiatrist, start reading my Bible, and that I was much better off than Christopher Reeve.

People with grief, hopelessness, and despair, need love, a little light in the tunnel, a hug and some proper pain relief. Mine had been present for several years and were due to an irregular heart beat, a pacemaker that did not work, difficult and painful urination, chronic leg and back pain, burning and painful feet, difficulty sleeping, inability to sit or drive a car, food intolerance, abdominal pain plus constipation, side effects of medication, and depression as well. I had stopped working, discontinued volunteer activities, avoided going to church and other social functions. I had Bob Dole's disease, stopped running, was avoiding my friends and family, had difficulty writing my name, and spent 80% of my time flat on my back or in bed. Over a five-year period, I had seven operations, a stroke, shingles (herpes zoster), chronic prostatitis and skin cancer. I became addicted to Ativan, narcotics, Darvoset, and sleeping pills, and in addition, took three different medications required for atrial fibrillation. I saw twenty-five different physicians and only one gave me the correct diagnosis. He confirmed that my depression was due to my disease, but not causing it. *And finally, I found out I had sensory peripheral neuropathy—as well as autonomic neuropathy.*

From the Internet, my daughter found out about the Neuropathy Association and my life began to change.

Soon I no longer had a death wish. As I improved, like John Senneff, my goal became to help others. God gave me a gift to make sick people more comfortable and He apparently had saved me to use that gift. From the Neuropathy Association I found out that many others had had the same experience. I found out about many support groups throughout the country. I discovered that autonomic neuropathy existed and was a major part of many of my ailments.

In September after seeing a Boston neuropathy specialist, who provided no additional help, I ordered a copy of the book *Toes and Soles.* (I had found out about it before from a fellow neuropathy patient.) That book tells it like it is and after reading chapters one and two, I had no doubt about the cause of my pain. It is difficult to relate all the vital and good things the information did for me. For example, I soon found out that the medicine I was taking was not helping me, but actually making me worse. I discovered which anticonvulsant medications to take and the proper doses. I added some minerals and some herbs. I have heeded the caution to use small or moderate doses of all medications. I learned about the other medical therapies to discuss with my neurologist and fortunately have not needed them. I have practiced relaxation and biofeedback and when I have difficulty urinating, I use patience and say the Lord's Prayer and after three times, it usually works. I found out that rest alone was killing my muscles and killing me, so now I exercise an hour a day. My diet of too much meat, dairy products, and sweets was destroying my stomach, digestion, and function of my colon, so now I am on lots of fruits and vegetables and fish. I don't dare touch chocolate, caffeine, sweets, or red meat and I've added Fibercon to my diet. Because of *Toes and Soles,* I had started taking some vitamins and after reading *this* book, I find that I need more. Both books do a good job of focusing on experimental and unapproved drugs plus new material that is in the works.

I am in the process of starting a support group for others with neuropathy who live in my area. *Toes and Soles* will be my Bible and my first textbook. For those picking up this book, you would be well advised to read *Toes and Soles* first. The present book, *Toes and Woes,* is a compendium on pain and the ways to control it. It could and should be a textbook for anyone treating persons with pain and certainly all patients who have peripheral neuropathy and autonomic neuropathy. Any medical specialist, whether he be a foot doctor or a head doctor, who sees patients with neuropathy, certainly should have both books in his office.

The content of *Toes and Woes* is well organized and I will try to briefly discuss each subject. Pain management with drugs and nutrient supplement is the meat of the book. Anticonvulsants are recommended as the mainstay for pain relief (I take two, Neurontin and Klonopin).

My pharmacist prepares a very effective topical agent for my feet, and topical agents are well discussed in chapter two. We are brought up to date on many physical types of medical therapies, most of which I hope I will never need. When I read chapter four on nutrients, I wanted to run to the health food store, because it seems that I need to take a few more. Some seem to be a must, especially for autonomic neuropathy. I definitely wanted to try ALA and increase my vitamin B-12 to a daily use and try a different type of Thiamine.

I am using some of the alternate/complementary therapies discussed in chapter five and plan to try more such as massage, meditation, and music therapy. Going to church regularly, attending a bible study group, and thanking God every day for my blessings and His help, is the least that I can do for the improvement that I have achieved. For the past four years, literally hundreds of members of my church have prayed for me, so I appreciate the elaboration on and the help from intercessory prayer.

Certainly no other medical person or academic researcher has compiled such a list of experimental therapies or future drug possibilities that are revealed in chapter six. Most are of the 21st century and are news to me, but they give all of us with peripheral neuropathy more hope. I particularly enjoyed chapter seven, entitled other matters. I have had herpes, experienced tic bites, scraped gallons of lead paint, used many cans of paint remover, and had my share of sports and running injuries. I have also taken Rythmol and Macrodantin. Both of these drugs can cause peripheral neuropathy.

All doctors should have a little touch of cancer, heart disease, or neuropathy. They should all have to take at least one or two "anti" drugs to know what it is like to be a patient. I could have written it, but our author has well discussed the subjects of finding a doctor, working with your doctor, getting a second opinion, and most importantly looking out for yourself and your loved ones. Our lives and our quality of lives are at stake.

In closing, I can't say enough good things about both books. My journey with my diagnosis is only one year old and the goal to start a support group in my community will be reached soon. I will use both books to educate others and to help my loving wife and family, who I live for; I will take a book to my psychiatrist; I will continue my Bible study; and I will continue to think about and pray for everyone like Christopher Reeve and all the other patients who suffer from peripheral neuropathy.

Richard D. Marks, Jr., M.D.
Mount Pleasant, South Carolina

Preface

Since the first publication of *Numb Toes and Aching Soles: Coping with Peripheral Neuropathy* (referred to as *Toes and Soles* here) in July 1999, readers have sent us hundreds of letters and "Request for Continuing Information" forms (included at the back of that book). There is a recurrent theme in these messages: many PNers (the term I then gave to all of us who have this obnoxious disease or, more properly, this "nerve disorder") are surprised to find they are not alone and that there are so many others in the same boat.

Indeed this boat is loaded with passengers. According to the Neuropathy Association, there are upwards of 22 million Americans carrying the unwelcome baggage called peripheral neuropathy.

That is an amazing number when you think about it—fifty times more than those diagnosed with multiple sclerosis, a much better known ailment! Of course, not all with PN experience severe pain or are disabled by it to the extent of so many with MS. Yet in the United States alone, more than two million lives are seriously compromised by peripheral neuropathy, according to some investigators.

Since *Toes and Soles* was published I have noticed a growing awareness that PN isn't all in the head, that it really *is* in the toes and feet, and sometimes in the hands, or occasionally in muscles that don't work as they used to. In other words, more and more non-PNers understand we PNers aren't crazy. (Any more than they are.)

Consequently we don't have to contort our faces in pain to show we're hurting. Or, lest we fear others will overlook our plight, gasp for air when we whisper we have peripheral neuropathy. (Just kidding, of course.)

Simply put, there seems to be an increasing realization that this strange thing we call peripheral neuropathy is not some kind of psychological aberration or cop-out from real-life responsibilities, but a serious problem that affects a lot of people. This growing recognition increases chances that sufficient research muscle (i.e., dollars) will be used to develop a cure.

Toes and Soles was intended to be a broad coverage of the entire subject of peripheral neuropathy—causes, symptoms, tests, treatments, new drugs in the pipeline, and coping strategies. There is no intent here to plow through the same ground, but I have dug deeper into the turf where new information warranted it. (If a particular drug or nutrient supplement, or a specific alternative or experimental therapy, is not further discussed here, be assured that I had not forgotten having written about it in *Toes and Soles,* but rather that no new development of interest or importance was found concerning it.)

This new book is focused on **treatments,** especially

treatments providing for **pain relief.** (Perhaps pain *amelioration* is a better term since neuropathic pain is hardly ever totally relieved.) I have emphasized pain relief because most PNers have the type of neuropathy known as "**sensory polyneuropathy,**" which produces various pain symptoms that are sometimes quite severe. These may include **aching, burning,** or **lancinating** or **tingling pains**—mainly in the feet or hands but sometimes in the legs or other parts of the body.[1] (**Autonomic** and **motor neuropathies** can be associated with pain and several treatments for these syndromes are also mentioned.)[2]

In fact, the principal goal for most people with PN—after they have in some cases spent a good deal of time and money looking for the **cause** of their ailment—is

---

[1] Of course there are many other words sometimes used to describe pain. The following are taken from the McGill Pain Questionnaire (MPQ): flickering, quivering, pulsing, throbbing, beating, pounding, jumping, flashing, shooting, pricking, boring, drilling, stabbing, lancinating, sharp, cutting, lacerating, pinching, pressing, gnawing, cramping, crushing, tugging, pulling, wrenching, hot, burning, scalding, searing, tingling, itchy, smarting, stinging, dull, sore, hurting, aching, heavy, tender, taut, rasping, splitting, tiring, exhausting, sickening, suffocating, fearful, frightful, terrifying, punishing, grueling, cruel, vicious, killing, wretched, blinding, annoying, troublesome, miserable, intense, unbearable, spreading, radiating, penetrating, piercing, tight, numb, drawing, sqeezing, tearing, cool, cold, freezing, nagging, nauseating, agonizing, dreadful, and torturing. Happen to find any of these that fit?

[2] Autonomic neuropathies affect involuntary or semi-voluntary functions such as control of the inner organs, sweating, constipation and bowel movements. Motor neuropathies concern such bodily changes as muscle weakness or atrophy, or cramps or spasms.

pain or other symptomatic **relief.**[3] (Of course if a cause is found that *can* be removed, or which will point to a particular treatment modality, great.)

You will also discover in this book that a few things well accepted by the medical community just a couple of years ago, "ain't necessarily so now." And, chances are, you might come upon a few completely **new ideas.**

In the end you will see there are few absolutes in dealing with peripheral neuropathy. Some of the studies you will read about are contradictory and reach opposite conclusions. Moreover, as was said repeatedly in *Toes and Soles,* what works for one may not work for someone else.

I know all this can be perplexing but the point of this book and *Toes and Soles* is to arm you with as much **information** as possible so that you can work with your doctor in adopting the best **treatment strategy** for yourself. (We need to hope he or she will be as well informed as you after you've read both books!) Talking about doctors, one of the more erudite said we are dealing with "therapeutic armamentaria" here. (But if you hear someone trying to impress you with a fancy term such as that, grab your hat.)

On the subject of treatments you will note that, because of funding priorities, most of the reported studies

---

[3] Peter James Dyck, Professor of Neurology at the Mayo Clinic, wrote in an editorial in *Archives of Neurology* (1999 May; 56{5}), that "often an underlying cause cannot be diagnosed with certainty; therefore, the emphasis must be on the treatment of pain, which is the main problem of patients with CSPN [chronic cryptogenic-cause unknown-sensory polyneuropathy]." The same thing we are talking about here.

concern **diabetic neuropathy.** The question arises as to the applicability of conclusions for these neuropathies to neuropathies of other known etiologies (i.e., causes)—or occurring in that great universe called **idiopathic** (cause unknown) neuropathies. Often times one can assume that, at least concerning **pain treatments,** there should be a great deal of **correlation** since the nerve or myelin damage which triggered the pain, regardless of the cause, is the same.[4] If the question, though, is correcting **other symptomatic aspects** or **neurological deficits** not strictly related to pain, or where a diabetic neuropathy could simply have been alleviated by **better glucose control,** or where the **mechanism of action** which caused the neuropathy can be identified and differs from other possible mechanisms,[5] the answer may not be the same. (It has always been surprising to me that so little attention has been directed to this matter of treatment correlation.)

By the way, in addition to "**allopathic modalities**" (another fancy medical term—this one referring to conventional medicine), special emphasis has been placed

---

[4] See the article "Pain in Generalized Neuropathies," by Arthur K. Asbury, M.D. (Professor of Neurology at the Univ. of Pennsylvania—and incidentally a contributor to *Toes and Soles*) in which he says that ". . . particular patterns of nerve fiber damage, regardless of how the damage is incurred, will result in neuropathic pain." From *Pain Syndromes in Neurology* (Butterworths 1990).

[5] Just one example here: people with diabetes may have particular trouble converting linoleic acid to GLA, as discussed later. Studies concerning GLA supplementation may be especially relevant for them.

here on **alternative** and **supplementary therapies,** particularly **nutrient supplementation.** I have become a firm believer, based on my own experience, in the proposition that **vitamins, minerals,** and certain **other nutrients,** can go a long way toward stabilizing or reducing (dare I say negating?) the effects of our peripheral neuropathies. I have obtained the thinking of several others who write frequently about nutrient supplementation and their ideas are set forth in this book.

As indicated in *Toes and Soles,* there is still **no true cure** for peripheral neuropathy. By this is meant the complete restoration of our peripheral nervous system—the repair and healing of the nerve axons and their protective myelin coating—to its original state, and the relief of all our neuropathy symptoms, so that we are just as before. However, progress continues to be made along this line and is discussed in this book. (Do not give up hope! They're working out there.)

I will add this as a personal note, for whatever it's worth. Four years ago I was in such pain in my feet I could hardly walk. We were making a house move at the time and I could not move a box from our car to our new home without taking a couple of time-outs on the path. Once we had moved in I didn't want to take my feet off a foot vibrator, which gave some (but temporary) relief. On a scale of 0 to 10, I would have rated my foot (feet?) pain at the time about an 8+ (0 being "Let's go dancing after we finish our tennis match" and 10 being, "God, I'm ready—please come get me, I can't walk over to you"). Now I'd give it about a 2—not non-existent but something I just don't think about all that much. (Now as far as my back is concerned. . . .) What I've done, which has made all the difference in the world, can be summed up with: the right **E**xercise, the right **M**edication, and the right nutrient **S**upplementation. (*Toes and Soles* had some fun with acronyms; EMS here definitely doesn't stand for Emergency Medical Service.)

My main purpose in this book, as in *Toes and Soles,* is to give you, if you are a PNer, the best and latest thinking on things you can do to achieve a better quality of life. If you are a family member or other caregiver whose lot is to take care of or at least be around somebody like us, I hope these two books will give you a greater appreciation of what your PNer is going through. If you are a medical professional called on to treat someone with peripheral neuropathy, I hope they will give you not only an understanding of what your PN patient is experiencing, but perhaps some new insights into our "disorder" and the possibilities for its treatment.

A final note. I am not a doctor, just a PNer like most of you reading this. (I have been in the PN corps for about 18 years now. If I had a calling card to send along with this book it would say "retired lawyer.") Once again, nothing herein should be taken as medical advice. You should consult a medical professional in connection with any therapy you intend to use, nutrient or otherwise, to make certain it is appropriate in your own case, with no unacceptable side effects for you. Your regular physician (if you have one, and you should) often is in a unique position to know your medical condition and how you've responded to particular medications in the past as well as how you are likely to in the future.

John Senneff
July 2001

P.S. I have attempted here to loosely follow the organization of *Toes and Soles* to facilitate cross checking on the reader's part. The idea is to let you compare the material chapter by chapter if you wish.

Incidentally, you may note many more full references to various studies than appeared in *Toes and Soles.* (Several doctors indicated to me they would like to have been able to get to the original source of more studies in the first book. Maybe they thought I made that stuff up?) Originally I intended to add these as endnotes in a bibliographic section under Roman numerals at the back of the book—to keep them separate from content footnotes numbered arabically and keyed to the associated body text—until I saw the awkwardness of anyone having to check citations borne on long Roman numerals—e.g., clxviii. Thus content footnotes and bibliographic references are all together on the relevant pages.

You will see content footnotes have been used rather extensively. There was much material I wanted to include for you that I thought was important or at least of collateral interest, and did, but I was trying to avoid interrupting the flow of the text as much as possible and not run a lot of incidental information into the main body of the book. Hopefully all these footnotes will not be too overwhelming. If they are, just keep your eyes focused above the horizontal lines at the bottom of the pages—unless your curiosity really gets you. Okay? I hope so.

Chapter 1

Neuropathic Pain—Further Insights

Chronic pain is often defined as that which lasts more than six months. (The following definition from the International Association for the Study of Pain may be more meaningful for many people: "Chronic pain syndrome is a condition in which pain has substantially interfered with a person's ability to function in normal life roles, and has eroded the pain sufferer's self-esteem, well-being, and relationships.")[1]

This kind of pain is fast becoming the number one medical complaint in America. According to the June 1999 issue of *Health After 50,* for example, as many as half of older Americans are plagued with persistent joint, muscle, or nerve pain.

Unlike pain protective in nature (for instance, pain caused by placing a bare foot suddenly on a hot pavement

[1] The following statement might get a ditto from many PNers: "Pain from [sensory neuropathies] can produce greater disability than the primary disease processes themselves." Robbins et al, *Anesthesia and Analgesia* (1998 Mar; 86(3): 579–83).

which prompts you to see how high you can jump),[2] chronic pain syndromes serve no useful purpose and once established, do not easily go away. In the case of **neuropathic pain,** for example, the subject continues to hurt as long as his or her brain receives pain signals from frayed or exposed nerves.

These neuropathic pain signals are often the result of **erratic firing patterns** emanating from the site of the nerve injury or from along the nerve fiber. The resulting paroxysms of pain can be stabbing or shooting, or in the case of numerous nerve fibers firing pain signals asynchronously (i.e., randomly), they can be burning.[3] (Just to review a bit, peripheral neurons are generally classified as **motor, sensory,** or **autonomic,** and most neuropathies are identified in the same manner. **Sensory neurons,** whose dysfunctions give rise to the type of neuropathies with which *Toes and Soles* and this book are mainly involved, are sub-classified into those with either **large-diameter** or **small-diameter fibers.** The large fibers primarily convey sensations of numbness and vibratory sensations such as tingling while the small fibers transmit temperature sensations and pain.)

---

[2] Of course if you have peripheral neuropathy, it's possible that you just might not feel a thing and leave your foot right there—no problem—till you see the 2nd degree burn marks on your sole! By the way, the hot foot example is what is referred to as nociceptive pain, the kind of reflex pain which, in medicalese, "stimulates the primary sensory nerves following a mechanical or thermal event."

[3] The strange anomaly of numbness co-existing with pain is due to the fact that some of the nerve fibers have died.

Two new technologies have enabled us to learn a good deal more about neuropathic pain over the last few years. Using **special imaging techniques,** researchers can now observe the manner in which pain signals travel through the peripheral and central nervous systems.[4] Also, scientists have been able to test the efficacy of new compounds in laboratory experiments by using specially bred **animals** which have been **genetically altered** to experience pain in much the same manner as humans. For example, a rat model with nerve injuries might have a super-sensitive reaction to a hair tapped on its hind-paw and will quickly pull it away. Some humans with neuropathic pain demonstrate a similar reaction; the light brush of a finger on the affected area can sometimes translate into extreme pain.

---

[4] Presentations at the Annual Meeting of the American Pain Society in early November of 2000 in Atlanta Georgia, showed how the use of single-photon emission computed tomography (SPECT), positron emission tomography (PET) scanning, and functional magnetic resonance imaging (fMRI), has led to a greater understanding of the pain experience.

To take one example of how these technologies are applied in current medical practice, consider the following from a recent study of acupuncture as a means to relieve pain: "Modern neuroimaging methods (functional MRI) confirmed the activation of subcortical and cortical centers, while transcranial Doppler sonography and SPECT showed an increase of cerebral blood flow and cerebral oxygen supply in normal subjects." *Wien Med Wochenschr* (2000; 150(13–14): 278–85). Another example directly involving peripheral neuropathy was presented by Dr. M. K. Yu at the University of Utah Health Sciences Center, who had reviewed a case where a woman with normal hematologic parameters was determined to have PN through cervical magnetic resonance imaging (*American Journal of Hematology,* 2000 Sept.; 65(1): 83–4).

In addition to the mimicking of pain reactions in humans, the use of animal models in clinical research permits the efficient testing of large numbers of agents for their painkilling effects in a shorter period.

(It should be recognized that animal work has its limitations, though. Dr. J. D. Ward at the Department of Diabetic Medicine, Royal Hallamshire Hospital, Sheffield, England, for example, points out that studies of pain pathways for nerve damage in animal models may not necessarily "reflect the human situation."[5] He maintains that techniques such as **magnetic resonance imaging (MRI)** will allow "more significant investigation of the human subject."[6] It would seem caution would be well advised in extrapolating from animal studies too freely.)

---

[5] There may be questions as to whether the study of nerve damage in animals even reflects the *animal* situation! An English investigation pointed out streptozotocin (STZ)-induced diabetes in rats has been increasingly used as a model of painful diabetic neuropathy to assess the efficacies of potential analgesic agents. The investigators wondered whether the resulting hyperalgesia (lowered pain threshold) was genuinely indicative of peripheral neuropathy or "may rather be attributed to the extreme poor health of the animals." According to the investigators, "indicative of their poor health, diabetic animals showed markedly reduced motor activity." *Pain* (1999 Jun; 81(3): 307–16).

The Merck Manual of Diagnosis and Therapy, Section 1, Chapter 4, had this to say in a different context: "[T]he relevance of animal studies of chromium deficiency to the effects of chromium in humans remains controversial."

The following observation seems particularly cogent: "Although animal models are helpful, they cannot take into account the emotions and other factors that affect human perception of pain." From "Treatment of Nonmalignant Chronic Pain," Dawn A. Marcus, M.D., University of Pittsburgh Medical Center, *American Family Physician* (March 1, 2000).

[6] *Diabetes Care* (1999 March; 22 Suppl 2: B84–8).

Toes and Soles referred to early work of Drs. Ronald Melzack and Patrick Wall in England. These pioneers found that pain signals are routed to the brain through the spinal cord and are temporarily stalled at a series of "**gates**" along the cord. Naturally occurring chemicals called **neurotransmitters,** which are the conveyors for the pain signals, collect at points called "**dorsal horns**" along side the spinal cord and remain there until the gates open. Once released these pain signals flock to the **thalamus,** the brain's pain center, where the pain is registered.

Much current work devoted to neuropathic pain relief is directed to suppressing these neurotransmitters. One way this can be accomplished is by **closing** the gates before the pain signals are ever released to the brain.

Neuropathic pain in reality is more complex than the foregoing discussion might indicate.[7] For example, one type of pain nerve can be **converted** into another under the influence of **chemicals** occurring in the body, leading to entirely **different** pain sensations. And as Dr. Ken McHenry of the International MS Support Foundation has said, with sufficient **stimulation** various types of pain nerves can be converted and aggregated at the same time to send ever more powerful pain signals.

Also the wiring of the nerves can be changed or "**reor-**

---

[7] Don't just take my word for it, see *Pain* (2000 Aug; 87(2): 149–58): "Peripheral neuropathic pain is produced by multiple etiological factors that initiate a number of diverse mechanisms operating at different sites and at different times and expressed both within, and across, different disease states." Not quite as easy as pie. (Or pi.)

ganized"—not only with respect to the sensory nerves directly affected by the nerve injury but also as to those in the spinal cord and even in the brain. Dr. Gary Bennett at the Allegheny University of the Health Sciences, maintains this reorganization helps account for the fact that certain drugs which are effective against normal or acute pain are unavailing against neuropathic pain, and vice versa.

Dr. Steven Richeimer of the Richeimer Pain Institute, says that animal studies suggest **abnormal electrical connections** can suddenly occur between adjacent nerves which are **demyelinated** (meaning their protective coating is gone). This so-called "**cross-talking**" may result in the **transfer** of signals from one nerve fiber to another. Other researchers have demonstrated that when large-diameter fibers, which carry feelings of vibration and touch (and for some PNers, tingling and "pins and needles" sensations) as previously mentioned, are damaged, so-called "**ectopic impulses**" can be generated in the small-diameter fibers which carry most pain sensations.

Another study, performed at Johns Hopkins and reported in the February 1999, issue of the *Journal of Neurophysiology,* demonstrated how neuropathic pain can leap from a nerve injury site to nearby skin, which can then become **exquisitively sensitive** to touch or temperature changes. Scientists partially severed a single pain nerve in an animal model and then examined the pain response in nearby, undamaged nerves leading to the skin. They found abnormal and spontaneous pain activity clearly indicated.

A study performed in Boulogne, France, also used animal models to demonstrate the complexity of neuropathic pain. The investigators found numerous **fiber interactions** following nerve injury, and even a number of changes induced in the central nervous system (the system comprised of the spinal cord and the brain, as contrasted with the peripheral nervous system which consists of all the other nerves in the body). They concluded that as the result of the "multiplicity of mechanisms," each of "the symptoms [of painful peripheral neuropathy] may correspond to **distinct mechanisms** and thus respond to specific treatments."[8]

In connection with the idea that different pain-producing mechanisms might be involved in PN, Dr. Hooshang Hooshmand, a leading authority on reflex sympathetic dystrophy (RSD—another important and disabling neuropathic disorder), observed in the *Pain Digest* that "simple **monotherapy**" is not sufficient. He said that treatment approaches should cut across several disciplines and use various modalities to deal with the frequently diverse pain mechanisms involved with neuropathic pain.[9]

(This requirement of multi-therapy approaches was seconded by presenters of various papers at the Annual meeting of the American Pain Society in Atlanta, Georgia, in early November 2000, where they considered the various neurobiologic and chemical pathways involved in

---

[8] *Acta Neurologica Scandinavica Supplementum* (1999; 173: 12–24).

[9] *Pain Digest* (1999; 9:1–24).

neuropathic pain syndromes such as diabetic neuropathy and reflex sympathetic dystrophy. The presenters noted that each of these syndromes probably entails at least several mechanisms, thus explaining the variable and usually incomplete response to any single therapeutic agent.)

Toes and Soles noted that many researchers believe there are **mixed psychological** and **physical aspects** to pain, and that there may be a direct relationship between chronic pain and emotions such as **fear** and **anxiety.** In light of that, a recent paper entitled "Fear and Anxiety: Divergent Effects on Human Pain Thresholds," seemed particularly interesting.[10] The authors pointed out that earlier animal studies had indicated that fear restrains pain whereas anxiety enhances it. They said, though, that it was not clear whether these outcomes are the same for human beings.

To delve into this matter the authors of the paper considered the effects of experimentally induced fear and anxiety based on exposure to, or the threat of exposure to, electric shocks. Based on the responses of 60 subjects randomized into different groups, the authors concluded that **fear** resulted in **decreased** pain reactivity, while **anxiety** led to **increased** reactivity, just as with animals. Both subjective and physiological indicators (skin conductance level and heart rate) confirmed these findings.

---

[10] *Pain* (2000 Jan; 84(1): 65–75).

Many PNers have said that when they first presented their pain complaints to their doctors, they were not given much help with **pain management.**[11] In some cases this might have been because the doctor was not sufficiently knowledgeable in dealing with neuropathic pain.[12] In others it could have been that the PNer was not accurately communicating the pain symptoms being experienced. Sometimes it might have been a combination of the two. Consider the following statement:

> A problem arises when chronic pain **feels** like acute pain, is described to (and is accepted by) physicians and

---

[11] I very much like this statement which appeared in an excellent paper on "Combining Analgesics for Better Pain Control," written by two pain experts at the University of Iowa College of Nursing: "The first priority of treatment is to treat the pain quickly and completely *as perceived by the patient* [my emphasis]. The second priority is to prevent a reoccurrence of the pain."

Concerning pain perception, how about the following "final word" from one pain expert: "Pain is what ever the experiencing person says it is, existing where ever the experiencing person says it does." Try getting your pain doc to buy that! (I submit he or she usually should.)

As of January, 2001, hospitals, nursing homes and out-patient clinics in the United States have been required to assess and treat a patient's pain just as any other symptom presented, or else risk losing their accreditation from the Joint Commission on Accreditation of Healthcare Organizations.

[12] A recent study in the journal *Neurology* reported that only 30% of neurologists surveyed believed they had been adequately trained to *diagnose* pain disorders and only 20% thought they were properly trained to *treat* them!

C. Peter N. Watson, M.D., in an article entitled "The Treatment of Neuropathic Pain: Antidepressants and Opioids," said that "Neuropathic pain is a common problem in patients seen by chronic pain specialists and is difficult to treat even in sophisticated hands." *The Clinical Journal of Pain* (2000 Jun; 16(2 Suppl): S41–48).

therapists as acute pain, and is then treated as acute pain. When this happens results are apt to be disappointing to both the patient and the physician and both may end up feeling quite frustrated. To both recover from, and to treat, chronic pain requires taking a different approach. However, most professionals, such as physicians, nurses, and physiotherapists, who are well trained in treating acute problems are not well trained in treating chronic problems. It will be up to you to find the appropriate professionals who do treat chronic conditions.[13]

Toes and Soles made the point that if a person thinks he or she might have peripheral neuropathy, a **neurologist,** and not just a general practitioner, probably should be seen at once; and not just any neurologist but one experienced in working with PN. However such a specialist might be hard to find, and even then might not necessarily be the best choice where very severe pain is involved.

As an alternative, there are many "pain clinics" which deal with pain exclusively, where PNers can go. The *Johns Hopkins Medical Letter* (June 1999) suggested a **multidisciplinary pain center** ought to be considered in many cases.

Such centers, typically affiliated with major hospitals or rehabilitation facilities, usually provide the type of total pain assessment and treatment suggested above by

[13] From "Self Help for the Chronic Pain Sufferer," The Victoria Pain Clinic. (undated)

Dr. Hooshmand for his RSD patients. Their operating premise is that pain is a **complex phenomenon** requiring input and expertise from a **number** of **medical disciplines.** These might include physicians from various specialties, physical therapists, psychologists, nurses and occupational therapists.

Often multidisciplinary pain centers will offer **non-traditional therapies** such as **acupuncture, relaxation techniques,** and **biofeedback,** in conjunction with conventional treatments. (These were all covered in *Toes and Soles* and will be further discussed here.) Although the experts at Johns Hopkins point out that total pain relief may not be possible, they claim most people participating in programs at these pain centers find significant improvement.

Incidentally, a Danish study investigated the differences in pain relief and quality-of-life outcomes experienced by patients treated at a multidisciplinary pain center versus those treated by a general practitioner who had been given initial supervision by a pain specialist.[14] One hundred and eighty nine patients with chronic non-malignant pain were studied. At referral, and after three and again six months, patients filled in questionnaires evaluating pain intensity, health-related quality of life and use of analgesics. After six months patients allocated to the pain center group reported "statistically significant" reductions in pain intensity, improvement in psy-

---

[14] *Pain* (2000 Feb; 84(2–3): 203–11).

chological well-being, quality of sleep and physical functioning. No improvements were seen in the other group. A reduction in the use of opioids administered on demand also was observed in the pain center group. The investigators concluded that, compared with the help obtainable from a multidisciplinary pain center, the establishment of a pain diagnosis and management plan by a pain specialist was not at all sufficient to enable the referring general practitioner to manage patients with severe chronic pain.

An article which appeared in the *Detroit Free Press* a while back provides some ideas on how best to find a pain specialist or pain center:

> Finding a good pain specialist isn't easy, but there are ways to identify doctors and medical centers with the most expertise.
>
> A center may have accreditation through the Commission on Accreditation of Rehabilitation Facilities (CARF) or the American Academy of Pain Medicine (AAPM). Doctors also may hold board certification in pain management or in a particular field, such as rehabilitation medicine. Board certification indicates that a doctor has passed national exams and stayed current in a field.
>
> Most pain centers describe themselves as multidisciplinary but vary in focus. Some are centered around a proven approach called functional restoration, a concept based on gradual increases in exercise or physical therapy, and behavioral-modification service and vocational rehabilitation.

In the end probably the best thing a PNer can do in finding a pain center is first, talk with a local doctor in whom you can place confidence and ask for help in locating a facility that might be suitable for your situation. When one or two have been identified, call one of them and ask to speak to the medical director. You might then ask about accreditation, methodological approach, staff, facilities, cost, etc. If a particular center appears of interest, it would be a good idea to make an appointment to visit the facility and, if possible, talk directly with a few of the professionals who would be working with you before you commit to their program. Remember always, you are in charge!

Before leaving the subject of pain, it should be noted that patients with sensory neuropathies—the type with which we are mainly involved here—often display **absent** or **reduced tendon reflexes,** or **slowed nerve conduction velocities.** As you will observe, in determining whether or not a particular therapy is helpful, a number of studies cited in this book focus on "**outcomes**" measuring those parameters—before and after treatment—in addition to **pure pain assessments.** In my opinion, though, whether a particular therapy is "successful" for *most* of us still comes down to the extent to which pain has or has not been reduced (putting aside autonomic and motor neuropathies, which have their own sets of associated horribles). It would be interesting to see more studies correlating such neurological abnormalities as slowed nerve conduction, reduced nerve fiber densities, and impaired temperature sensations, directly with pain.[15]

---

[15] In a paper, "Measurement of Nerve Dysfunction in Neuropathic Pain," the statement is made, "Neuropathic pain is difficult to diagnose and treat. Both can be made easier if the nerve dysfunction can be quantified." *Current Review of Pain* (2000; 4(5): 388–94). That appears to beg the question. The author of the following statement at least recognizes there may be a correlation problem: "*Presumably*, the combined finding of improved nerve function and improved nerve morphometry [physical measurement] will predict improvement in long-term clinical outcomes such as impaired sensation, *painful neuropathy,* insensitive feet, neurotrophic ulceration, and/or amputation. *However, data to support this possibility are still lacking* [my emphases]." *Diabetes* (1995; 44: 1355–61).

Chapter 2

Pain Medications: New Studies, New Thinking

One can properly surmise from the headings of the first four sections of this chapter—"Antidepressants," "Anticonvulsants," "Antiarrhythmics" and an "Antispasmodic"—that the medications discussed in each were originally designed for rather different purposes than dealing with peripheral neuropathy. Fortunately (for us), these various drugs often have beneficial effects for our malady and are frequently prescribed for PN. Here we update the information in *Toes and Soles* to the extent that there have been significant new studies performed or new insights gained concerning currently prescribed pharmaceuticals. Also included are discussions of a few medications not mentioned in that book which have recently been used for the treatment of peripheral neuropathy.[1]

---

[1] Many medical professionals employ a "ladder approach," devised by the World Health Organization originally for cancer, for various

Antidepressants

Antidepressant medications are sometimes classified into four categories: **monoamine oxidase inhibitors; tricyclics; serotonin reuptake inhibitors;** and **heterocyclics.** We are primarily concerned with the second category, tricyclics, although a couple of the serotonin reuptake inhibitors and one of the heterocyclics may hold promise for us.

1. Tricyclics

The **tricyclic** antidepressants (**TCAs**) are often prescribed as the initial therapy for the management of neuropathic pain.[2] In fact **Elavil** (amitriptyline), **Norpramin** (desipramine), **Pamelor** (nortriptyline), and

---

kinds of chronic pain. The first ladder step for mild-to-moderate pain involves the use of acetaminophen, aspirin, or another NSAID combined with an adjuvant agent—a drug that has other indications but is analgesic in specific circumstances.

Patients with **moderate-to-severe pain** are treated with an oral opioid combined with a non-opioid analgesic as well as an adjuvant drug. In the treatment of continuous pain, analgesics are given on a regular basis—"by the clock"—so that the next dose is given before the effect of the previous one wears off.

Pain that is persistent or **severe** is treated by increasing opioid potency or using higher dosages. Drugs such as codeine or hydrocodone are replaced with more potent opioids (usually morphine, hydromorphonet methadone, fentanyl, or levorphanol). Medications for persistent pain are administered on an around-the-clock basis, with additional as-needed doses.

[2] *Neurology* (2000; 55 (5 Suppl 1): S41–6; discussion S54–8). "Tricyclic" means a chemical with three rings, usually fused, in the molecular structure.

Tofranil (imipramine), are considered by some doctors to be the weapons of choice.[3]

In a paper delivered to the Peripheral Nerve Society in July 1999, "Drugs for Pain in Polyneuropathy, How Effective Are They?" the authors ranked tricyclic antidepressants as the "most effective" class of medications.[4] The findings presented there by Dr. S. H. Sindrup at the Department of Neurology in the Odense and Aarhus University Hospitals in Demark were further amplified in an article following that meeting which appeared in an issue of *Pain*.[5] There he said, concerning various studies:

> We identified all placebo controlled trials and calculated numbers needed to treat (NNT) to obtain one patient with more than 50% pain relief in order to compare the efficacy with the current treatments, and to search for

---

[3] Ibid., 915–20.

[4] In a paper presented to the Annual Meeting of the American Pain Society in early November 2000, in Atlanta, Georgia, the author, Zahid H. Bajwa, M.D., said that, "Based on clinically and statistically significant randomized, controlled studies, gabapentin [to be discussed] and tricyclic antidepressants seem to be most efficacious in the treatment of painful diabetic neuropathy and postherpetic neuralgia." He added, though, that "none of the studied antidepressant or antiepileptic agents has provided complete analgesia [pain relief] as a single agent for any of the above neuropathic pain syndromes."

A review in the journal *Drugs* concluded that although TCAs as a class are the agents of choice for painful diabetic neuropathy, they are ineffective in approximately 50% of patients treated and are generally not well tolerated." (1998 Oct; 56(4): 691–707). (Look on the bright side. This means they must be effective 50% of the time! Actually some other studies show a more favorable ratio than this. *Toes and Soles* reported studies that indicated *60%* of patients get 50% or more pain relief from TCAs. That up's it a bit.)

[5] *Pain* (1999 Dec; 83(3): 389–400).

> relations between mechanism of pain and drug action. In diabetic neuropathy, NNT was 1.4 in a study with optimal doses of the tricyclic antidepressant imipramine as compared to 2.4 in other studies on tricyclics. The NNT was 6.7 for selective serotonin reuptake inhibitors, 3.3 for carbamazepine, 10.0 for mexiletine, 3.7 for gabapentin, 1.9 for dextromethorphan, 3.4 for tramadol and levodopa and 5.9 for capsaicin. . . . In peripheral nerve injury, NNT was 2.5 for tricyclics and 3.5 for capsaicin. . . . There were no clear relations between mechanism of action of the drugs and the effect in distinct pain conditions or for single drug classes and different pain conditions.[6] [Abstracted from the article.]

It seems that Dr. Sindrup is suggesting, for example, patients with diabetic neuropathies would have to take about four times as much mexiletine to accomplish the same result as tricyclics (10.0 versus 2.4), based on "optimal doses" of each. (He did add that some of the treat-

---

[6] Other studies and experience have suggested a relationship between specific drugs/drug classes, and particular "pain conditions," although certainly the relationship is not always clear. *Toes and Soles* ranked drugs in terms of the type of pain *primarily* addressed by each drug: either burning, or shooting/stabbing, or aching pains. It was, of course, recognized that certain pharmaceuticals might be useful for dealing with more than one kind of pain and were so classified. Some studies do not attempt any distinctions in this regard. A Medical Education Collaborative paper delivered late in 1999 for CME by Bennett et al., entitled, "Anticonvulsant Therapy in the Treatment of Neuropathic Pain," noted this failing. The authors, referring to a particular study, said in frustration, "This aspect of their study [concluding certain anticonvulsant drugs provided considerable relief for shooting or lancinating pain] makes it completely impossible to determine whether anticonvulsant drugs are only effective for shooting pain, are more effective for shooting pain than for other types of pain, or are equally effective for neuropathic pain regardless of its specific quality."

ments other than tricyclics may be important due to their better tolerability.) One conclusion that can surely be drawn from Dr. Sindrup's study is that **imipramine** is the **most effective** among the tricyclics.

A study review focused specifically on the question of whether all tricyclic antidepressants are equally effective in the treatment of painful diabetic neuropathy, was undertaken by Dr. J. D. Joss at the University of Iowa. After running a search of "randomized controlled studies" covering the period from January 1966 to December 1998, she concluded simply that the **data** was **insufficient** to answer the question of superiority in efficacy. She did state that "**amitriptyline** and **desipramine** are **reasonable first choices** in treating diabetic neuropathy."[7]

Yet in a 1998 study, amitriptyline was found to be no more effective than **mexiletine** (trade name Mexitil[8])—a drug like the tricyclics often prescribed for burning

---

[7] *Annals of Pharmacotherapy* (1999 Sep; 33 (9): 996-1000).

[8] Some drugs are protected by patents and are supplied by only one company. These are known as trade-named or branded products. However, when the patent expires, other manufacturers can produce a generic version of the drug. Currently, about half the drugs on the market are available in generic form. On average, generic drugs are said to cost about 50% as much as their brand-name counterparts. For some drugs, the savings are reported to be as much as 90%. (I must be going to the wrong pharmacies.)

Most state laws provide that a generic drug be *generically equivalent* to its brand-name counterpart. That is, it is required to have the same active ingredients, strength, and dosage form—pill, liquid, or injection. *Toes and Soles* pointed out, however, that the generic form may not always have the same standard of "bioavailability"—the amount of medication entering the patient's circulatory system and becoming available therapeutically. Because of that and perhaps because of occasional personal biases, some neurologists and other medical practitioners prefer prescribing brand-name medications to pains—and neither were found to be significantly more effective than placebo! The study was a randomized, double-blind, placebo-controlled,[9] 10 week trial of 145 patients with HIV-associated peripheral neuropathies in which the primary outcome measured was **pain intensity.**[10]

Amitriptyline fared no better than acupuncture in another randomized, "modified" double-blind, trial. This one involved 250 patients with HIV-related peripheral neuropathy and was conducted at centers in 10 different cities. Once again, placebo proved just as good as amitriptyline in relieving pain; acupuncture was found no more useful.[11]

---

generic products even when the latter are available. As the patient, however, you can always tell your doctor you want the *most effective* drug at the best price, and you can ask him or her to write prescriptions for generic drugs when available meeting your requirements.

At the time this was written a few major drug manufacturers who have built their businesses on their branded products have, interestingly, begun themselves to offer generic products. In part this is believed motivated by criticism that these companies are profiting excessively from high prices on their branded products. (Nationwide branded products accounted for 59% of prescription fulfillments in 1999 but about 91% of prescription costs.)

[9] "**Randomized**" means the study participants are assigned to groups in such a way that each participant has an equal chance of being assigned to either the treatment or to the control group. Since randomization ensures that no specific criteria are used to assign any patients to a particular group, all the groups will be equally comparable. (At least that's the idea.) "**Double-blind**" means neither the investigator nor the subject knows which medication (or placebo) the subject is receiving. "**Placebo**" is an inactive substance or sham therapy designed to resemble the drug or therapy being tested. It is used as a control and is designed to hopefully rule out any psychological effects testing may present.

[10] *Neurology* (1998 Dec; 51(6): 1682–88).

[11] See *JAMA* (1998 Nov 11; 280(18): 1590–95).

New studies continue to show that when relief from neuropathic pain is obtained from tricyclics, the relief is **independent** of their **antidepressant properties** *per se.* (See, e.g., McQuay H, Moore RA, *An Evidence-Based Resource for Pain Relief,* Oxford University Press 1998.) *Toes and Soles* had made a similar point—patients who benefit from tricyclic antidepressants experience pain relief before any uplift in mood.

2. Selective Serotonin Reuptake Inhibitors (SSRIs)

An antidepressant which was first approved by the FDA in 1993 for the treatment of depression and anxiety is now generating new interest in the treatment for neuropathic pain. **Venlafaxine** (trade name **Effexor**) was briefly mentioned in *Toes and Soles,* together with several other non-tricyclics which all are strong **selective serotonin reuptake inhibitors (SSRIs).**[12]

A study was reported in *Diabetes Care* in 1999 in which venlafaxine was given to 10 patients with diabetic neuropathy, each of whom had been treated unsuccess-

---

[12] Based on then current thinking, the statement was made in *Toes and Soles* that "In the past they [SSRIs] have been aimed more at counteracting depression than for pain relief." Obviously this statement now must be modified.

SSRIs in general act to boost the levels of the neurotransmitter, serotonin—which sends messages to and from the brain—by blocking the neuron reuptake pumps. (The reuptake pumps are used by neurons to recycle neurotransmitters previously released into the synaptic cleft—a gap between neurons. By blocking these reuptake pumps, SSRIs make more neurotransmitters available in the fully with other medications. When the drug, at a dose of 37.5–75 mg per day was administered, all patients reportedly had a 75–100% reduction in pain within 3–14 days. No side effects were observed.[13]

Results of another study involving 244 non-depressed diabetic outpatients 18 years of age or older who were randomly assigned to treatment with venlafaxine or a placebo for up to 6 weeks were presented in July 2000, to the 60th Scientific Session of the American Diabetes Association in San Antonio, Texas. Overall, venlafaxine was reported to have provided significantly better pain relief compared with placebo. Higher doses of venlafaxine (150 to 225 mg daily) significantly decreased pain intensity compared with placebo and with lower doses (75 mg daily). In fact at the end of the sixth week, 56% of patients receiving venlafaxine at the higher doses reported significantly decreased pain intensity versus 39% of patients receiving the 75 mg regime and 34% who were treated with placebo.[14] Because patients with depression were excluded from the trial, symptomatic improvement was ascribed solely to the **pain-killing effect** rather than any antidepressant action.

---

synaptic cleft, and through successive neurotransmissions, to the brain. The result is that pain perception is reduced.) As a drug class SSRIs offer the advantage of having fewer side effects than the tricyclics. Venlafaxine increases the levels of both the neurotransmitters serotonin and norepinephrine in the brain. These two neurotransmitters are involved not only in the perception of pain but also the mediation of mood.

[13] *Diabetes Care* (1999 Nov; 22(11):1909–10).

[14] The so-called "placebo effect" is well known. On average it is said that one third of subjects in a clinical trial will report significant

Nausea was the most common side effect. Others that may occur with use of this medication are said to include insomnia, nervousness, anorexia (loss of appetite), and weight loss, as well as blood pressure increases.

Another SSRI, **paroxetine** (trade name **Paxil**), was found in two earlier studies to be potentially useful in treating diabetic neuropathy. In the first, the drug was tested against **imipramine** (a tricyclic) and placebo in a randomized, double-blind, cross-over trial.[15] Paroxetine was given as a fixed dose of 40 mg per day, while the dose

---

improvement simply from a sugar pill. To demonstrate that a treatment is effective, it must be shown that it performs significantly better in the treated group as opposed to the control or placebo group.

In spite of the "placebo effect," placebos have long been used in clinical studies as the best way of determining whether a new therapy has a consequence on the disease or illness it is intended to treat. Under the rules of informed consent, subjects must be told in advance of a study concerning placebo use and that they may be among those who receive it. Whether a person receives the agent being tested or a placebo depends on chance, and only after the conclusion of the study will anyone know who was in each group.

In an article written November 27, 2000, entitled "Placebos: Deceptive Benefits," for CNN Health, Jeffrey P. Kahn, Ph.D, Director at the Center for Bioethics, University of Minnesota, said:

> "The only problem with this approach is that prospective subjects often don't appreciate the fact that they may be in the placebo group. Studies have shown that the vast majority of subjects believe that they will be put into the research group that is best for their treatment. But researchers don't prejudge what's best for subjects, and if every subject received what was perceived to be in his or her best medical interests, research would be very difficult to conduct. *Of course it may be the case that those in the placebo group do better—not because the placebo has more therapeutic effect, but because it has fewer side effects than the drug being tested* [my emphasis]."

[15] *Pain* (1990 Aug; 42(2): 135–44). In a **cross-over** trial each patient is in each group at different times.

of imipramine was adjusted to yield optimal plasma levels of imipramine. Paroxetine was found to have significantly reduced the symptoms of neuropathy as measured by both clinical observer—and self-rating, but was somewhat less effective than imipramine. The investigators suggested by dose adjustment, though, that paroxetine may become as effective as imipramine. The investigators also noted that five patients who were on imipramine dropped out because of intolerable side effects and four of 19 completing the study reported withdrawal symptoms after discontinuing imipramine. No patients dropped out who were on paroxetine due to side effects, and no withdrawal symptoms were reported.

The other study was a review of paroxetine's "pharmacology, therapeutic use in depression, and potential in diabetic neuropathy."[16] Noting that paroxetine has shown "potential in the symptomatic treatment of diabetic neuropathy," the investigators said that in older people with major depression, short term (six weeks) treatment produces clinical improvements "significantly superior to placebo and similar to those with tricyclic antidepressant agents." They also noted that paroxetine offers an important potential advantage over the tricyclics in the setting of overdosage; in the latter case overdosage can lead to more serious adverse events.

A more recent study dealt with the effect of paroxetine on neuropathy in a tangential way.[17] It noted that after

---

[16] *Drugs and Aging* (1993 May-Jun; 3(3): 278–99).
[17] *American Heart Journal* (2000 Oct; 140 Suppl(4): 77–83).

myocardial infarction, an abnormal reduction in beat-to-beat **heart rate variability** (a measure of **cardiac autonomic innervation** by the brain) is a strong predictor of death. With loss of innervation to the **vagus nerve** (a nerve that principally supplies the viscera with autonomic sensory and motor fibers), as is noted in patients with **severe neuropathy** and in heart transplant recipients, there is loss of heart rate variability. The study then noted that although tricyclic antidepressants reduce heart rate variability, treatment with paroxetine normalizes it.

According to an article by Dawn A. Marcus, M.D., University of Pittsburgh Medical Center, entitled "Treatment of Nonmalignant Chronic Pain," (*American Family Physician,* March 1, 2000), the use of the SSRIs, **sertraline** (**Zoloft**), 150 mg once a day, and **paroxetine** (**Paxil**), 30 to 70 mg once a day, can reduce neuropathic pain by 70 to 80 percent.

A "systematic review" focused on the SSRIs in general found, after looking at the results of 19 studies, that three of the SSRIs were effective for "mixed chronic pain," but that it was "unclear whether they are beneficial for tension headaches, migraine, *diabetic neuropathy,* and *fibromyalgia* [my emphasis]."[18]

3. A Heterocyclic

Trazodone (trade name **Desyrel**) is another antidepressant, by type designated a **heterocyclic** (this term

---

[18] *General Internal Medicine* (1997 Jun;12:384–89).

refers to its chemical structure), which has received some recent recognition for treating diabetic neuropathy. In a somewhat similar fashion to the SSRIs (to which, however, it is not chemically related), trazodone works by **inhibiting the uptake** of two neurotransmitters, **serotonin** and **norepinephrine.**

In a study of 31 patients with painful diabetic neuropathy, 19 reportedly experienced symptomatic relief and 7 experienced complete relief after two weeks of therapy.[19] (Eight patients discontinued the drug because of side effects, but they were considered relatively minor—insomnia, headache, and dizziness.)

The Mayo Clinic in an article, "Managing Pain," indicates that trazodone is one of the antidepressants which "may offer some relief for people with chronic pain, whether or not they also have depression." The article points out that trazodone (together with the antidepressant tricyclics) "is especially useful for neuropathic, head and cancer pain."[20]

Jack D. McCue, M.D., Professor of Medicine at the University of Massachusetts Medical School, says that heterocyclic antidepressants are especially helpful in elderly patients with pain. According to Dr. McCue: "Small doses of trazodone or doxepin may be particularly useful in improving sleep in these patients."

Miles J. Belgrade, M.D., at the Sister Kenny Institute & Abbott Northwestern Hospital in Minnesota, notes

---

[19] *Journal of the American Podiatric Medical Association* (1999 Sep; 89(9): 468–71).

[20] *Mayo Clinic Health Letter* (June 10, 1999).

that trazodone has the advantage of **fewer side effects** and a **better safety profile** than the tricyclics.

4. The Score for Antidepressants

An important study considered the effectiveness and safety in general of antidepressants in neuropathic pain. In a systematic review of randomized controlled trials,[21] the investigators reported that, "Compared with placebo, of 100 patients with neuropathic pain who are given antidepressants, 30 will obtain more than 50% pain relief, 30 will have minor adverse reactions and four will have to stop treatment because of major adverse effects."[22] The investigators added that, "With very similar results for anticonvulsants it is still unclear which drug class should be first choice." (It will be recalled from earlier discussion that for 50–60% of those taking tricyclics—one category of the antidepressants—there was said to be a 50% re-

---

[21] *Toes and Soles* reported that anyone interested in forthcoming clinical trials should bookmark the web site, *www.centerwatch.com.* Early in 2000 the National Library of Medicine's ClinicalTrials.gov site was launched and as of the time this was written, had data on 5200 trials. For the most part these were sponsored by the National Institutes of Health. The Library plans to add trials sponsored by other federal agencies, pharmaceutical companies, and by others in the private sector. (Note: To find current studies of interest to PNers, I suggest you do a search at the ClinicalTrials.gov site on "neuropathy" as well as on "neuropathy, peripheral" and "neuropathy, diabetic," using commas as indicated. If you are interested in considering participation in a particular trial which is recruiting, there is usually a contact person listed.)

[22] *Pain* (1996 Dec; 68(2–3): 217–27).

duction in pain—a more optimistic outcome than the foregoing study would suggest for antidepressants as a whole.)

Anticonvulsants

In general, anticonvulsants are thought to decrease neural membrane excitability and to increase the threshold for activation. Probably the first anticonvulsant commonly prescribed for neuropathic pain was **carbamazepine,** also referred to by its trade name, **Tegretol.** (Actually the very first drug may have been diphenylhydantoin. Its use was reported 60 years ago for **trigeminal neuralgia,** or "tic douloureux.")[23]

Carbamazepine is used today to treat TN,[24] an extremely painful disorder involving compression of the trigeminal root, as well as to treat other neuropathic syndromes involving "**electric shock**" or **stabbing type pains.**[25] It is still the only drug which carries an FDA-approved indication for neuropathic pain. (The other drugs currently being prescribed for peripheral neuropathy have been approved by the FDA only for other ail-

---

[23] *Rev Laryng* (1942; 63).

[24] In a recent Finnish study of TN induced in small animal models, baclofen was found superior to carbamazepine in treating **allodynia** (hyper-sensitivity to touch) behavior. The allodynia behavior had been found resistant to morphine and also to amitriptyline. (*Pain* 1999 Feb; 79 (2–3); 281–90).

[25] See Fields HL, *Pain* (New York: McGraw-Hill; 1987).

ments. Their use for PN is called an "off label" application, which is permissible under the law.)[26]

1. Gabapentin (Neurontin)

The leading and seemingly most prescribed drug for neuropathic pain in the anticonvulsant category—or probably in any category—is **gabapentin** (trade name **Neurontin**).

Pre-clinical studies of this pharmaceutical for PN had been suggested by anecdotal reports in the mid 90s, showing that it seemed to be effective in dealing with complex regional pain syndrome (a.k.a. reflex sympathetic dystrophy or RSD). Since the studies on Neurontin reported in *Toes and Soles,* new ones have underscored its usefulness.

In a randomized, double-blind, placebo-controlled eight week trial reported late in 1998, gabapentin "monotherapy" was assessed. The drug was titrated (gradually increased) from 900 to 3600 mg daily (up to the maximum tolerated) for 84 patients who had a one to five year history of pain attributed to diabetic neuropathy. Placebo was administered to 81. The investigators examined the patients' mean pain scores at the end of the study and reported they were significantly lower for the gabapentin

---

[26] For years the FDA has affirmed the properness of these uses. In a letter to the Pain Research Group at the University of Wisconsin Medical School dated 9/28/94, Stuart L. Nightingale of the FDA wrote: "The agency has long recognized physician's use of drugs outside the approved labeling within the context of the practice of medicine."

group than for the placebo group. They also reported that "all secondary outcome measures of pain" were significantly better for the gabapentin group.[27] In concluding remarks they said "gabapentin monotherapy appears to be efficacious for the treatment of pain and sleep interference associated with diabetic peripheral neuropathy and exhibits positive effects on mood and quality of life."[28]

The most common "adverse events"[29] during the trial were somnolence (19.3 percent versus 8.7 percent with placebo); dizziness (17.1 percent versus 6.9 percent with

---

[27] Measuring pain and analyzing pain scores is a science unto itself. First there are various so-called single dimension pain scales. These include the "numerical pain scale" (0 representing "no pain" and 10 "worst pain"), the some what similar five-point Likert scale, and the "visual analog scale" (i.e.,VAS—using a 0 to 10 line with the patient making a mark somewhere along its length). Then there are multi-dimensional scales such as the McGill Pain Questionnaire (MPQ) which combines various measures such as a pain rating index, an indication of "present pain intensity" on a scale of 1 to 5, and patients' selections from a host of verbal descriptors. (See fn 1 of Chapter 1.) There also are techniques of behavioral analysis and analyses based on patients' graphic depiction choices or patients' use of and reliance on medications. But it can get much more complicated. Consider the following from a study on the synergistic effect of combining amitriptyline and electrotherapy for pain relief:

> "Wilcoxon's rank sum test was used for analyzing changes in pain scores. The percentage of improvement in symptoms was analyzed by Student's *t* test. Statistical calculations were performed using Dyna-stat Professional Statistics Software (Dynamic Microsystems, Washington DC) on an IBM personal computer." *Diabetes Care* (1998 Aug; 21(8): 1322–5).

[28] *JAMA* (1998 Dec 2; 280(21): 1831–36). Also reported in *Epilepsia,* (1999; 40 Suppl 5:S57–9; discussion S73–4).

[29] The term "adverse event" can have a formal and specific significance. In an FDA drug trial it includes "any injuries by overdosing, abuse/dependence, and unintended interactions with other medicinal products."

placebo); ataxia (an inability to coordinate voluntary muscular movements—12.5 percent versus 5.6 percent with placebo); fatigue (11 percent versus 5 percent with placebo); nystagmus (a rapid, involuntary oscillation of the eyeballs—8.3 percent versus 4 percent with placebo); and tremor (6.8 percent versus 3.2 percent with placebo).

Following JAMA's publication of this study, the lead investigator, Dr. Miroslav Backonja, Associate Professor of Neurology at the University of Wisconsin Medical School and a well-known pain specialist, said in an interview that, "Gabapentin is a very welcome addition to our options for pain control. It is well-tolerated by most patients and stands apart from other drugs in that it doesn't interfere with other medications." He also noted that gabapentin does not interact or compete with other substances, an important consideration for diabetics who frequently must take several medicines.[30]

In another study reported in JAMA late in 1998, gabapentin was tested for the treatment of "postherpetic neuralgia" (PHN), a syndrome of often intractable neuropathic pain. The study was a multi-center, randomized, double-blind, placebo-controlled investigation involving 229 subjects. In a four-week titration period, up to a maximum of 3600 mg of gabapentin or matching placebo was given daily. The primary efficacy measure was change in average daily pain scores. Secondary measures were

[30] Dr. Backonja was back on ja scene a few years later, authoring a paper which was published in the *Clinical Journal of Pain* (2000 Jun; 16(2 Suppl): S67–72) on "Anticonvulsants for Neuropathic Pain Syndromes." He reaffirmed his support for the efficacy of gabapentin, and said it "should be a first-line treatment for neuropathic pain."

average daily (perhaps it should have been called average nightly?) sleep scores. Subjects who received gabapentin had a reduction, which the investigators called significant, in average daily pain score from 6.3 to 4.2 points compared with a change from 6.5 to 6.0 points in subjects randomized to receive placebo. Secondary measures of pain as well as changes in sleep interference showed improvement with gabapentin. The investigators concluded that "gabapentin is effective in the treatment of pain and sleep interference associated with PHN. Mood and quality of life also improved with gabapentin therapy."[31]

However, gabapentin had a little wind taken out of its sails in San Diego in 1999. There the drug was pitted head-to-head against amitriptyline in comparing efficacy for treatment of diabetic neuropathy. The randomized, double-blind study included 28 participants, half given average daily doses of 1565 mg of gabapentin and half given average daily doses of 59 mg amitriptyline over a six week period. The findings announced at the end of the study were that "although both drugs provide pain relief, mean pain score and global pain score data indicate no significant differences."[32] The investigators made a point in saying that gabapentin was more expensive than amitriptyline. (That was still true at the time this was written because gabapentin remained under patent and was being marketed as Neurontin while amitriptyline is available in a generic form. In fact *Toes and Soles* indi-

[31] *Clinical Journal of Pain* (1998 Dec 2; 280(21): 1837–42).
[32] *Archives of Internal Medicine* (1999 Sep 13; 159(16): 1931–37).

cated a cost difference for a typical daily dose, of about 10 to 1 between the two.)

There was a return match staged in Italy between the two drugs the following year. (Clearly amitriptyline gets into many frays.) In a 12-week, randomized, open label (no placebo) trial, 25 patients with diabetic neuropathy were divided into two groups, one receiving gabapentin titrated up to 1200 mg per day and the other amitriptyline titrated from 30 mg to 90 mg each day. The trials lasted 12 weeks, the initial doses being increased over a 4 week period and the maximum doses administered for 8 weeks. Measuring pain intensity and *paresthesia* (sensations of numbness, tingling, etc.) intensity, the investigators concluded that not only did gabapentin produce greater reduction in pain and *paresthesia,* but "adverse events" were less frequent in the gabapentin group than in the amitriptyline group.[33]

Incidentally, a paper entitled "Gabapentin Use in Neuropathic Pain Syndromes," examined the complex changes and events which take place in the peripheral nervous system following the onset of peripheral neuropathy.[34] These include the release of intracellular calcium ions, the unblocking of the magnesium ion plug on the NMDA (N-methyl-D-aspartate) receptor, and the initiation of protein kinase C activation. (Aren't you glad you asked?) The author, Dr. B. Nicholson at the Lehigh Valley

---

[33] *Journal of Pain and Symptom Management* (2000 Oct 1; 20(4): 280–85).

[34] *Acta Neurologica Scandinavica* (2000 Jun; 101(6): 359–71).

Hospital Pain Center in Allentown, Pennsylvania, said that "gabapentin may interrupt an entire series of events, not just a single process, that lead to the development of neuropathic pain." He went on to say that gabapentin "effectively antagonizes the maintenance" of "inflammatory and neuropathic pain." (The Bennett paper, "Anticonvulsant Therapy in the Treatment of Neuropathic Pain," previously mentioned in a footnote, refers to several studies reporting that gabapentin was effective in ameliorating a wide range of pain syndromes, including burning, shooting, throbbing, and cramping pain. In fact, it was the only drug listed in *Toes and Soles* as dealing with all of the neuropathic pain types.)

In conclusion, among the various medications used to treat peripheral neuropathy, gabapentin seems to be considered by more doctors and by more patients as the **most effective drug** for PN, with the least objectionable side effects and the least unwelcome drug interactions. As a study in *Drugs* maintained, "Based on the positive results of these studies [referring to various trials] and its favorable adverse effect profile, gabapentin should be considered the first choice of therapy for neuropathic pain."[35]

This is still not to say that gabapentin is the best medication for *all* PNers. It does not work for everybody and the side effects, even if generally considered acceptable for many, are intolerable for some.

---

[35] *Drugs* (2000 Nov; 60(5): 1029–52) Gabapentin seems to have more "first choice" proponents than any or all the tricyclics or other antidepressants taken together in spite of statements such as appeared in an earlier paper published in *Drugs*—see footnote 24 above.

2. Lamotrigine (Lamictal)

Another anticonvulsant discussed in *Toes and Soles* in the chapter on "Experimental or 'Unapproved' Drugs," can be put, with some reservations, in the "current treatments" column now.

Lamotrigine (trade name **Lamictal**) primarily acts on the **central nervous system** to control the number and severity of **seizures.** As a "voltage-sensitive sodium channel blocker" and inhibitor of the release of the neurotransmitters, **glutamate** and **aspartate,** it is thought to depress the activity of certain parts of the brain and to suppress the abnormal firing of neurons that causes seizures. It generally is taken in conjunction with other anticonvulsants.

Toes and Soles mentioned results of a lamotrigine study presented to a Neuroscience of HIV Infection meeting in Chicago in June 1998. The full study was reported in *Neurology* in June 2000.[36] The drug had been initiated at 25 mg per day and slowly titrated over seven weeks to 300 mg daily. Of the 42 enrollees with HIV-related neuropathies, 29 finished, with 20 receiving placebo and 9 lamotrigine.[37] At the end of the 14-week study period the

[36] *Neurology* (2000 Jun; 54: 2115–19).

[37] Of the 13 who dropped out, 11 were in the lamotrigine group, a relatively high percentage, and of those, 5 left because of rashes. Rashes such as those experienced can be quite dangerous. In fact one out of 1000 adults who take the drug reportedly come down with Stevens-Johnson syndrome, a potentially fatal condition. (This is a rare disorder characterized by inflammation of the mucous membranes of the mouth, throat, anogenital region, intestinal tract and membrane lining the eyelids.)

average reduction in pain was about three times greater in the lamotrigine group than in the other. The investigators said that the pain reduction was "equivalent to a decrease from moderate to less than very mild pain," and was "clinically significant." However "peak worst pain" was similar for the two groups.

Two other studies in 1998 reached similar conclusions. In an open trial conducted to study the potential efficacy of lamotrigine on diabetic neuropathy, dosages beginning at 25 mg daily were titrated up to 400 mg/day over six weeks. Fifteen patients began the trial with two dropping out before its conclusion due to "adverse effects." By various measures pain scores dropped about in half for those finishing it. The investigators concluded that lamotrigine was "potentially effective and safe in treating painful diabetic neuropathy."[38] In the other, lamotrigine was tested on just two patients. The English investigators concluded that the drug "can be used to treat neuropathic pain," although they called for double-blind, placebo-controlled studies to substantiate their findings.[39]

The following year other English investigators did that, conducting a randomized, double-blind, placebo-controlled trial in which 74 patients were given doses increasing to 200 mg/daily. At the end of eight weeks the investigators concluded (rather remarkably based on the earlier studies) that, *at the dosage used,* lamotrigine

---

[38] *European Journal of Neurology* (1998 Mar; 5(2): 167–73).
[39] *Anaesthesia* (1998 Aug; 53(8): 808–809).

had no effect on pain sensitivity, numbness, *paresthesia,* sleep, mobility or quality of life.[40]

In an interesting study performed in Belgium in 2000, 20 patients with "chronic, neuropathic pain not responding to interventional therapy," were tested.[41] Lamotrigine was administered either as a **monotherapy** or in combination with **oral morphine.** Ten patients were said not to have responded at all while four were "temporary responders" and six reportedly sustained longer term pain relief. The investigators said that the combination of lamotrigine and morphine in particular produced "excellent pain relief for more than five months" and they hypothesized an additive effect between the two.

Finally, in a wrap-up late in 2000, Irish investigators reviewed all the "accumulating evidence" indicating "that lamotrigine is effective in the treatment of neuropathic pain."[42] In their report they indicated they had considered the "molecular action of lamotrigine in terms of its effects in pre-clinical models of pain and hyperalgesia" and said the literature suggested that it "may be effective" in the management of neuropathic pain.

3. Topiramate (Topomax)

A relatively new anticonvulsant, **topiramate** (trade name **Topamax**), is also being used by some physicians

[40] *Pain* (1999 Oct; 83(1): 105–107).

[41] *Journal of Pain and Symptom Management* (2000 May; 19(5): 398–403).

[42] *Clinical Journal of Pain* (2000 Dec; 16(4): 321–26).

for treating their PN patients. This medication was approved by the FDA in 1997 for the adjunctive treatment of adults with partial-onset seizures. Although the precise mechanism of action is unknown, one theory suggests that its anticonvulsant activity may be due in part to increasing **GABA** (gamma-aminobutyric acid), a neurotransmitter that inhibits excitation of nerve cells in the brain. In trials it appeared to be more potent than gabapentin or lamotrigine for antiepileptic purposes.[43]

An article in *Primary Psychiatry* (August 1999) entitled "Topiramate Treatment of Neuropathic Pain," discussed the case of a sixty-year old man with shooting pains who had tried the whole gamut of pharmaceutical treatments, including all the TCAs, gabapentin, mexiletine, carbamazepine, and lamotrigine. According to the article, after six months with a regimen of 50 mg of topiramate in the morning and 75 mg at night, he experienced 80% relief "around the clock without intolerable side effects."

A pilot study of topiramate in the treatment of painful peripheral neuropathy was reported to the Peripheral Nerve Society in July 1999 involving 19 patients. At the time this book was being written results had not been released. Dr. David R. Cornblath at the Johns Hopkins University School of Medicine, told me that a large placebo-controlled, multi-center study was being planned.

In a somewhat related study, Michael Haugh, M.D.,

---

[43] *Medical Sciences Bulletin* (1997 Feb; 20(1)).

and Gregory Connor, M.D., from the Headache and Neurological Center in Tulsa, Oklahoma, conducted a retrospective analysis of eight patients at their center who had been treated with topiramate for trigeminal neuralgia.[44] These patients had experienced pain from one to 16 years, and five had been treated unsuccessfully with other drugs, including gabapentin, carbamazepine, phenytoin, and baclofen. Four patients taking topiramate monotherapy and two taking topiramate plus carbamazepine reported good to excellent pain relief. (Two patients discontinued topiramate because of nausea and dizziness, and another for personal reasons.)

Topiramate is usually given at 50 mg a day in the beginning, with titration to 400 mg daily, divided into two doses. Adverse effects are said to include psychomotor slowing, difficulty in concentration, speech problems and fatigue.[45] Also topiramate may interact adversely with phenytoin (Dilantin) or carbamazepine (Tegretol), according to reports; both of these medications are sometimes prescribed as peripheral neuropathy treatments.

---

[44] Program and Abstracts of the 19th Annual Scientific Meeting of the American Pain Society; November 2–5, 2000; Atlanta, Georgia. Abstract 675.

[45] An interesting study was undertaken at the University of Alabama at Birmingham Epilepsy Center, Department of Neurology, assessing the cognitive effects of gabapentin, lamotrigine, and topiramate. After the administration of these three drugs to separate groups of "healthy young adults" over a four week period, the investigators found more significant declines in measures of attention and word fluency for the topiramate group than for the other two. *Neurology* (1999 Jan 15; 52(2): 321–27).

Antiarrhythmics

Two oral **antiarrhythmic** drugs, used mainly to treat **cardiac dysfunctions,** have occasionally been used in the treatment of neuropathic pain: **mexiletine** (trade name **Mexitil**) and **tocainide.** The latter, however, reportedly has more side effects and is not often prescribed for this purpose.

Mexiletine, an **oral analog** of **lidocaine** (an anesthetic used by dentists), blocks sodium channels and therefore inhibits transmission of impulses along injured nerves. It has about a 15 year (off-label) history in treating peripheral neuropathy, particularly in Europe.

The first known study in which mexiletine was used for painful diabetic neuropathy was performed in Denmark in 1988. Sixteen of nineteen patients were assessed in a randomized, double-blind, cross-over trial following the daily administration of 10 mg/kg bodyweight of the drug. Using a five-item clinical symptom scale, the researchers found "significant improvement during the mexiletine phase as compared with the placebo phase."[46]

Three years later Ackerman et al., opined that oral mexiletine could be "considered with those patients whose diabetic neuropathy is resistant to more conventional forms of treatment."[47]

---

[46] *The Lancet* (1988 Jan 2–9; 1 (8575–76): 9–11).

[47] *Journal of the Kentucky Medical Association* (1991 Oct; 89 (10): 500–501).

Stracke et al., gave a strong endorsement to mexiletine in 1992[48] and again in 1994[49] studies. The latter was a double-blind, placebo-controlled, multi-center investigation. Pain responses were evaluated for 95 patients with painful diabetic neuropathy who had received 450 mg of mexiletine daily (for an unstated number of days). The investigators said the patients who would benefit most from mexiletine therapy were those with "stabbing or burning pain, heat sensations, or formication." (Careful there!—formication just means those creepy-crawly sensations, as if you can't get those pesky flies off your face, your legs, or your whatever.) They also noted that efficacy did not seem to rise "proportionally" with dosage increases. One interesting sidelight was a statement that mexiletine proved a "very safe therapy with negligible side effects, *even less than placebo* [my emphasis]." (It makes you wonder what they laced the placebo with!)

The lack of side effects was again mentioned in a study reported in 1995 in Japan, where researchers found "remarkable pain effectiveness" for five patients suffering from "painful alcoholic neuropathy," with particular relief noted from "tingling and aching sensations." The researchers found the minimum effective dose to be 300 mg of mexiletine daily.[50]

Reports from a Swedish study two years later were that the drug not only appeared to reduce pain caused by

---

[48] *Diabetes Care* (1992 Nov; 15(11): 1550–55).
[49] *Medizinische Klink* (1994 Mar 15; 89(3): 124–31).
[50] *Internal Medicine* (1995 Jun; 34(6): 577–79).

diabetic neuropathy, with "no serious adverse events," but that it seemed to have "a rapid onset."[51]

The validation road began to get rocky for mexiletine that same year, based on a study performed at the University of Kansas Medical School. Wright et al. performed a double-blind, randomized study with 29 patients, giving 600 mg daily of mexiletine or matching placebo for three weeks. They found no "statistically significant" difference in pain scores between mexiletine and placebo following the conclusion of the study. The investigators said that "this drug should be reserved for patients unresponsive or intolerant to standard therapy, without evidence of heart disease, and with sensations of burning heat, formication (there's that word again), or stabbing pain."[52]

Further questions were raised in a 1998 study at the Santa Clara Valley Medical Center in San Jose, California. Twenty-two patients with HIV-related peripheral neuropathy were randomized to receive mexiletine (maximum dose, 600 mg daily) or placebo for six weeks. Again, no statistically significant difference was found in mean daily pain scores between the two groups at the end of the study. Importantly, dose-limiting adverse events occurred in 39% of those receiving mexiletine.[53]

A review was conducted in New Zealand that same year of various trials in which mexiletine had been used

---

[51] *Diabetes Care* (1997 Oct; 20(10): 1594–97).

[52] *Annals of Pharmacotherapy* (1997 Jan; 31(1): 29–34).

[53] *Journal of Acquired Immune Deficiency Syndromes and Human Retrovirology* (1998 Dec 1; 19(4): 367–72).

for painful diabetic neuropathy. The reviewers noted that the frequency of adverse events in patients receiving mexiletine in these trials ranged from 13.5 to 50%. They said that gastrointestinal complaints, particularly nausea, were the most common. The reviewers relegated mexiletine's status to "an alternative agent for the treatment of painful diabetic neuropathy in patients who have not had a satisfactory response to, or cannot tolerate, tricyclic antidepressants [their first choice] and/or other drugs."[54]

In looking back at these studies and reviews, I am struck by the diversity of reported results—particularly the receding perception of efficacy and the increasing uneasiness about side effects over time.[55] It is almost as if somebody had switched the formula in the mid 90s. After pondering this material, my own "un-doctored" view is that mexiletine would not be the first drug I would want to take for my (idiopathic) PN and only if nothing else were working would I *consider* trying it.

An Antispasmodic

The drug **baclofen** (trade name **Lioresal**), discussed in *Toes and Soles* as a **muscle relaxant** and **antispas-**

---

[54] *Drugs* (1998 Oct; 56(4): 691–707).

[55] Mark S. Wallace, in an article, "Calcium and Sodium Antagonists for the Treatment of Pain," (*Clinical Journal of Pain,* 2000 Jun; 16(2 Suppl): S80–85), also took note of the differences in reported efficacy between earlier and later studies. He said that "it appears mexiletine is a poor choice for the management of neuropathic pain with a prominent allodynia [again, the phenomenon in which normally inoffensive stimuli causes pain]."

modic (also occasionally referred to as an **antispastic**), is sometimes prescribed for neuropathic pain. Generally it seems to be used only after other drugs have been tried. **Tizanidine** (trade name **Zanaflex**) was also mentioned in T*oes and Soles* as a muscle relaxant that is less often administered for neuropathic purposes. Similarly to baclofen, it acts on the central nervous system to produce its effects.

Recently there has been renewed interest in tizanidine for treating neuropathic pain. An article in mid-1999 mentioned the drug among "several promising new medications" for dealing with trigeminal neuralgia, a disorder of unilateral facial pain characterized by lancinating paroxysms of pain in the gums, lips, cheek or chin.[56] The authors noted that carbamazepine (also discussed in *Toes and Soles*) had been considered the standard first-line treatment for years.

In late 2000, an open label (unblinded) study was conducted to consider tizanidine's effectiveness and tolerability (the latter sometimes being a major issue with baclofen) for neuropathic pain relief.[57] One to four mg of tizanidine was administered daily for one week to 23 patients, titrated weekly thereafter until a maximum of 36 mg, or the patients' tolerability limits, were reached. (The mean dosage was 23 mg/daily.) Weekly pain scores and the frequency and severity of adverse events were observed.

---

[56] *Archives of Family Medicine* (1999 May-Jun; 8(3): 264–68).
[57] *The Journal of Pain* (2000 Winter; (1)4).

Average pain scores had decreased by about 25% at the end of the study period, with 15 patients (68%) reporting their pain relief had "improved or much improved," and two reporting complete pain relief. Side effects consisted primarily of dizziness/lightheadedness (52%), drowsiness (48%), fatigue/weakness (43%), dry mouth (39%), gastrointestinal upset (30%), and sleep difficulty (22%). The researchers concluded that tizanidine "might be an effective treatment for neuropathic pain, offering an alternative for patients poorly responsive to other medications."

(Investigators in a study reported earlier that year concerning the use of tizanidine in the management of **musculoskeletal** complaints, maintained that the use of the drug **did not** result in the "debilitating muscle weakness [caused by] other antispasmodic agents."[58] They also noted that when the drug was taken at night, patients indicated it helped them in getting to sleep with little "hangover sensation" upon waking. The investigators concluded that "tizanidine is potentially helpful to many palliative care patients [i.e., patients whose symptoms are being treated, and where no cure is being sought] with **chronic muscle pain** and sleep disturbances.")

Tizanidine is usually taken several times a day. Medical practitioners advise patients not to take more than 36 mg in a 24-hour period. Too much of this medication can damage one's liver, they warn.

---

[58] *American Journal of Hospital Palliative Care* (2000 Jan; 17(1): 50–58).

Topicals

Topical treatments for peripheral neuropathy come in a variety of forms. Usually they are **creams,** which are semisolid emulsions of oil and water, easily applied, and which disappear when rubbed into the skin. As to other topical nomenclature:

- **Ointments** contain little if any water and generally feel greasy. Drugs in ointments are often more potent than in creams.
- **Lotions** originally were suspensions of powdered material (e.g., calamine) in a water or alcohol base; most modern lotions (e.g., some corticosteroids) are water-based emulsions. They are convenient to apply and often feel cooling and drying to the skin.
- **Solutions** are homogenous mixtures of two or more substances. Like lotions, solutions are drying, and especially easy to apply. The most commonly used bases are ethyl alcohol, propylene glycol, polyethylene glycol, and water.

Topical treatments are often favored because, being applied only to the surface of the skin, they do not result in significant increases in serum drug levels. Moreover, they tend not to cause interactions with other drugs or adverse systemic side effects.

1. Capsaicin

Toes and Soles dealt at length with a particular topical, generally sold in a cream form, called **capsaicin.** One of the most frequently used versions is a non-prescription product called Zostrix, available either in a .025 or .075% strength.

Capsaicin is a medication derived from **cayenne/red peppers.** Its mode of action is to deplete a peptide neurotransmitter called **substance P** from nerve endings so that pain impulses cannot be easily transmitted to the brain.

As indicated in *Toes and Soles,* most studies have shown capsaicin to be effective in the treatment of neuropathic pain. (However, because of the **burning sensations** it produces, many people cannot tolerate it for the four weeks or so believed to be required to achieve results.) A more recent study, though, casts some doubt on efficacy, at least with respect to HIV-related neuropathies.

In a multi-center, placebo-controlled, randomized and double-blind study, 26 subjects were enrolled and received either capsaicin or placebo.[59] At no time during the four-week trial did the investigators find any difference between the two groups with respect to "current pain, worst pain, pain relief, sensory perception, quality of life, mood, or function." They concluded (not unreasonably

[59] *Journal of Pain and Symptom Management* (2000 Jan; 119(1): 45–52).

based on those findings) that capsaicin "is ineffective in relieving pain associated with HIV-associated PN."

Another randomized, double-blind, placebo-controlled trial tested .025% capsaicin cream against 3.3% **doxepin** and against a combination of .025% capsaicin and 3.3% doxepin hydrochloride cream. The researchers said that overall pain was "significantly reduced" to the same extent in the groups taking the differing creams. They noted that the capsaicin cream "significantly reduced sensitivity and shooting pain," although burning pain was increased. They also noted that the capsaicin/doxepin combination produced **more rapid** pain relief than either alone.[60]

Incidentally, there was an interesting article in the April 13, 2000, issue of *HealthSCOUT,* reporting on work involving a nerve cell site called the "**capsaicin receptor.**" It appears that a molecule sits on the surface of the site and responds to specific chemical triggers by opening the cell to a flood of sodium and calcium. Dr. James Julius and colleagues at the University of California at San Francisco, who discovered the capsaicin receptor in the mid-1990s, developed a strain of mice that lacked the capsaicin receptors. They compared the pain responses of the mice with altered receptors to other mice, and found the former less sensitive to heat and pressure. Based on this work, Dr. Julius believes it may be possible to develop drugs that take advantage of the site's special

---

[60] *Journal of Clinical Pharmacology* (2000 Jun; 49(6): 574–79).

characteristics, particularly drugs to fight pain caused by inflammation.

2. Lidocaine

As previously mentioned, **Lidocaine** is an **anesthetic** used by dentists. It acts to block sodium channels, thereby inhibiting the transmission of impulses along injured nerves. The medication is often used in various topical applications to alleviate PN pain.[61]

A paper appeared in the June 2000 issue of the *Clinical Journal of Pain* concerning **lidocaine patches** manufactured by Endo Pharmaceuticals, Inc.[62] The author noted that these patches had recently been approved by the FDA for the treatment of **postherpetic neuralgia** (acute nerve pain caused by herpes) and added that studies had shown that they may be effective for "chronic neuropathic pain" as well.[63]

A study assessing the effectiveness of these patches appeared in the same journal several months later.[64] In

---

[61] *Toes and Soles* made the point that oral administrations of lidocaine are used as predictors of whether mexiletine, previously discussed, will be effective in dealing with neuropathic pain in particular individuals. Lidocaine also is used systemically as a direct therapeutic tool for PN. (*Pain,* 2000 Jul; 87(1): 7–17).

[62] They consist of a 10 x 14 cm patch with polyethylene backing and a medication-containing adhesive made up of 5% lidocaine (700 mg per patch) and several other ingredients such as water and glycerin. Lidoderms come 30 to a pack which reportedly sells for about $155–160.

[63] *Clinical Journal of Pain* (2000 Jun; 16 Suppl (2): S62–66).

[64] *Clinical Journal of Pain* (2000 Sep; 16(3): 205–208).

an open label investigation, 16 patients with refractory (resistant to treatment) PN pain were enrolled. They had variously reported intolerable side effects or inadequate pain relief with antidepressants, anticonvulsants, anti-arrhythmics, and opioid medications. The investigators found, from reviewing pain scores, that 13 of the 15 participants who completed the study experienced "moderate or better pain relief."

These patches, sold in the U.S. under the trade name **Lidoderm,** are reportedly available only by prescription.

3. Clonidine (Catapres)

Clonidine (tradename **Catapres**) is generally used for treating **hypertension.** In a gel form it also has been found to produce **localized analgesia** (i.e., pain relief).

Sherwyn Schwartz, M.D., and colleagues at Albert Einstein College of Medicine, Bronx, NY, studied the safety and analgesic effect of topical clonidine gel for the treatment of pain in 10 patients with chronic diabetic neuropathy.[65] A 0.05% clonidine gel was applied to feet or legs twice daily for the first two weeks. The dosing frequency was then gradually increased to four times daily until the end of the six week study.

Patients were evaluated at enrollment and at two, four and six weeks, rating their pain on a 10-point pain

---

[65] Program and Abstracts of the 19th Annual Scientific Meeting of the American Pain Society; November 2–5, 2000; Atlanta, Georgia. Abstract 671.

scale ranging from 0 (no pain) to 10 ("pain as bad as it could be").

At the end of the study, all reported some pain relief, with three patients claiming "complete relief" and seven "moderate relief." Adverse events were "mild."

4. Other Topical Combinations

There are also various topical preparations using **combinations** of ingredients for treating PN pain, usually in the form of a cream. *Toes and Soles* mentioned several, one involving **prilocaine** and **lidocaine** (**EMLA**), another **lidocaine** and **ketoprofen,** and still another, **lidocaine** with both **bupivacaine** and **indomethacin.**

Dr. Ed Davis, a podiatrist, said in a "Podiatry OnLine" forum in August 1999, that he has achieved a better than 70% success rate in the mitigation of pain associated with diabetic neuropathy with the following formulation: **2% amitriptyline** and **2% baclofen** in a "pluronic lecithin organogel" applied initially three times daily.[66] (Essentially this same formulation was mentioned in the December 1999 edition of the *Neuropathy News,* a publication of the Neuropathy Association.)

---

[66] He said that this "PLO" gel was highly lipophilic (meaning having an affinity for lipids such as fats) and allowed good percutaneous (through the skin) absorption of the active ingredients. Lecithin gels such as the one Dr. Davis uses reportedly have a number of properties which make them a desirable vehicle. They can be obtained with biocompatible components, are stable for extended periods, and can solubilize sizeable amounts of quite different chemicals.

Dr. Davis said that the 30% of patients who did not respond to that preparation were treated with the same formulation plus **1% ketamine.** He added that although the concentration of ketamine was at a low level (other formulations have used more), his results were "remarkable."

The same formulation has been used by Dr. Neil A. Burrell, DPM, CDE, who wrote in *Diabetes Interviews* (January 2000), that he applies the compound three times a day to feet where the neuropathic pain occurs, and that the treatment offers immediate relief. For "recalcitrant neuropathic pain," he writes, "many times we use a **combination** of **tramadol, gabapentin** and **amitriptyline.**"

Incidentally, a study was conducted to discover whether a topical application of ketamine in a PLO (gel) would relieve neuropathic pain without causing the usual unwelcome side effects of other forms of ketamine administration.[67] The result in five patients participating in an open study was significant pain reduction—on the order of 65 to 100%—with no reported side effects. Initial response was said to have occurred within 20 seconds to three minutes!

Dr. Robert Arvanaghi, an M.D. at the Pain Management Clinic Suburban Hospital in Bethesda, Maryland, uses a topical preparation of **10% lidocaine** and **20% ketoprofen** in many pain syndromes, including diabetic neuropathy. He says that he has used this preparation

---

[67] *Intl J Pharm Comp* (1998 Mar/Apr; 2(2): 122–27).

with dozens of patients who have had good results and that the side effects have been "essentially non-existent."

Dr. Robert Shackelford, an M.D. from Cushing, Oklahoma, has used a 5% PLO/NSAID gel applied directly to the affected area two to three times daily, and says he has achieved a success rate of "approximately 90%." He points out that **transdermal NSAIDs** have significant advantages over oral preparations since they do not produce gastritis.

A recent study suggested that a formulation of **desipramine** and **amitriptyline** could be beneficially developed as a cream or gel to deal with **inflammatory** neuropathic pain.[68] According to the investigators, such a formulation might achieve pain reduction "with limited systemic side effects."

5. Compounded Preparations

The pharmacists who prepare medications such as the foregoing, are called "**compounding pharmacists.**" They are specially trained to make custom formulations specifically meeting the prescribed requirements of patients.

This practice allows the physician to order a custom-tailored medication not available commercially. Also it permits pharmacists to prepare small quantities of a prescription more frequently to ensure stability of the product for its intended use. Still another—and to me more

[68] *Pain* (1999 Aug; 82(2): 149–58).

cogent reason in so far as treating our ailment is concerned—is that compounding permits the pharmacist to use two or more medications at the same time, substances which may work differently but have a synergistic effect when used in combination.[69]

Often a compounding pharmacist will use a **transdermal gel** (a form intended for absorption through the skin) as a base or vehicle for the topical application of the active ingredients. This permits the medication to be directed to the precise area where it's needed. The method reportedly reduces side effects or adverse events associated with the oral ingestion of some of the tricyclics, for example.[70] Transdermal administration is also said to help assure faster and more effective pain relief in many cases. Another attractive feature is that by combining various medications, **smaller concentrations** of each medicine can sometimes be used.

---

[69] Another *raison d'etre* for this profession is that drug manufacturers must be assured there will be a return on their investment before they come out with a new product. The result is that there are limited chemical forms, dosage forms, strengths, flavors and packaging available for the physician to prescribe, which can be severely restrictive for the practitioner. Compounding can solve this problem. For example, a patient may be allergic to a preservative or dye in a manufactured product that a compounding pharmacist can prepare in a dye-free or preservative-free form. Another example might be where a patient has difficulty swallowing a capsule and requires a troche (a type of lozenge which is placed between the cheek and gum to deliver active ingredients across the oral mucosa) prepared by the compounding pharmacist.

[70] "Topical non-steroidal anti-inflammatory drugs have a lower incidence of gastrointestinal adverse effects than the same drugs when they are taken orally." *British Medical Journal* (1998 Jun; 319: 331–38).

One of the better known compounding pharmacists in the country, Eric Everett (O'Brien Pharmacy in Kansas City, Missouri), told me that he has found a **combination** of **ketoprofen, clonidine** and **ketamine** for transdermal application to be especially useful in treating PN pain.

Incidentally, there is an organization called the **International Academy of Compounding Pharmacists,** with 1300 members. Their web site is http://www.iacprx.org, and their telephone 1-800-927-4227. By entering your zip or postal code at the place indicated on their web site, they will give you the name and address of local compounding pharmacists in your area.

It is important to remember that, as with any drug mentioned in this book, a doctor's prescription is required to obtain practically every medication ordered from or prepared by a pharmacy, whether compounded where you order it or supplied by a manufacturer.

Opioids (and a Near Opioid)

This section probably should be titled "**Narcotics**" except that there is so much prejudice and emotionalism attached to that word that most commentators use a softer word—"**opioids**"—almost as a euphemism. Technically, though, "opioids" are limited to **synthetic narcotics** such as **oxycodone, methadone** and **meperidine** while the broader term "narcotics" more properly includes all of those as well as drugs derived from opium (opiates), such as **morphine** and **codeine.** As you will see, I have followed the herd and use the "opioids" term to describe all of these substances since most of the studies and practically all the literature do so even when discussing substances which are really opiates. Incidentally, some of the writings in this area use the terms "**opiates**" and "opioids" interchangeably, without making a distinction between the two. (Confused? I'll say it all another way then . . . . On second thought, maybe that's enough.)

1. Uses and Reservations

Traditionally these "opioids" have only been prescribed for **chronic cancer** or **acute nociceptive pain** (the kind often following an injury). Many medical professionals have long taken the stance they are not useful in dealing with neuropathic pain.[71] This perception is beginning to change, however. Watson et al., reviewing therapies used in a number of "randomized, controlled trials," noted that "opioids are increasingly being used for the refractory patient."[72] The authors maintained that for these patients, "chronic opioid therapy may be the only avenue

---

[71] One earlier study, however, had suggested a more accommodating position, maintaining that "opioids should not be withheld [in the treatment of neuropathic pain] on the assumption that pain mechanism, or any other factor, precludes a favorable response." *Pain* (1990 Dec; 43(3): 273–86).

[72] *Pain Research and Management* (1999; 4(4): 168–76); *Clinical Journal of Pain* (2000 Jun; 16 Suppl (2): S62–66). Some clinicians still maintain that although opioids *may* be effective for neuropathic non-cancer pain in some instances, they are more effective for nociceptive pain. (See, e.g., *Drug Safety,* 1999 Oct; 21(4): 283–96).

of relief, and evidence is accumulating that this approach is safe if proper guidelines are observed."

According to an article in *Oncology News International,*[73] Dr. Richard Payne of the Memorial Sloan-Kettering Cancer Center, found that patients with pure neuropathic pain such as with diabetic neuropathy, experienced equally effective relief from either opioids or drugs more typically used for such purposes, e.g., gabapentin.

He believes that while **non-opioid analgesics** work quite well in reducing mild neuropathic pain, moderate or severe pain usually requires an **opioid drug,** often in combination with other drug therapy. He also made a distinction between **weak opioids** such as **codeine, dihydrocodone, meperidine,** and **oxycodone** in combination with **acetaminophen, aspirin,** and/or **caffeine,** and **stronger ones** such as **methadone, morphine, fentanyl,** and **oxycone** (in its sustained-release form). He said the stronger opioids can be used for moderate or severe pain at higher doses without toxicity concern,[74] and with no ceiling as to their efficacy, in contrast with the weaker ones employing **acetaminophen, aspirin,** and/or **caffeine** (!)[75]

---

[73] *Vol. 8, No. 6, June 1999.*

[74] "Opioid analgesics are the cornerstone of pharmacological treatment of moderate to severe pain." (From "Combining Analgesics for Better Pain Control," Duffy and Eland, University of Iowa College of Nursing.)

[75] Dr. Payne said that transdermal fentanyl (Duragesic)—covered in *Toes and Soles*—has become quite popular for chronic pain. He said it is released across a "rate-controlled membrane" for 72 hours,

A much more conservative approach to the use of opioids is evidenced in an editorial by Dr. Peter James Dyck, Department of Neurology at the Mayo Clinic, appearing in the May 1999 issue of *Archives of Neurology* (Vol. 56, No. 5), where he wrote in part:

> In my opinion, such drugs as morphine, meperidine, or levorphanol tartrate generally should not be used for treating painful neuropathy of the kind discussed herein [sensory polyneuropathy], because they are associated with excessive drowsiness (which is not compatible with a productive life over a long time) and because they predispose to habituation and addiction. However, there may be a place for the use of milder narcotic agents, such as codeine, oxycodone, and propoxyphene napsylate. For some patients with severe discomfort, low dosages of these agents may be prescribed with a reasonable benefit-risk ratio. Generally, these medications should be combined with another analgesic (e.g., aspirin or acetaminophen) and taken only when completely necessary (and usually toward the end of day or evening). Also, a certain daily upper limit should be set and adhered to. There is a definite need for regular medical surveillance to ensure that the set dosage of narcotics is not exceeded, that the need for pain relief is still present, and that the drug is not being used for pleasure (to get "high").

The modern view is trending towards a more accommodative role in the use of opioids. Increasingly, doctors

---

offering noninvasive, continuous, passive diffusion of the drug across the skin. He added that when a chronic pain patient is faced with breakthrough pain, there is an acute need for increased analgesia. That is "best dealt with through IV morphine or the new fentanyl lozenges [Actiq], which when mixed with saliva, penetrate the oral mucosa and reach therapeutic levels as fast as IV morphine," he said.

appear willing to use any or all of these substances when treating chronic pain where they feel the pain cannot be otherwise controlled. Before they tended to be more fearful that they could lose their licenses or face other legal consequences if they were accused of over-prescribing and contributing to drug addiction.[76] Their willingness to consider this strategy seems well supported by the fact that **true addiction** (psychologic dependency) is uncommon (reported to be between 5 to 15%), particularly where the opioids are **long acting.**[77]

In this regard it is sometimes pointed out that although the **short acting** types (e.g., **Percocet, morphine, Vicoden,** etc.) are useful for acute pain, they are also more associated with sedating and euphoric side effects. Further, their nature is believed to encourage their overuse and the development of tolerance (the need for increased dosages to achieve initial effects).

---

[76] As reported in *Toes and Soles,* many have believed the principal problem is not addiction but rather *under-prescribing.* How times are changing, though. The *New York Times* reported a recent case of a doctor in Oregon required by the Board of Medical Examiners to undergo retraining after failing to give patients *enough* opioids for pain control!

Several states have enacted "intractable pain" legislation which more clearly permits physicians latitude in prescribing opioids for non-cancer pain patients.

[77] An article on "Prescribing Opioids" by John F. Lauerman, a medical writer, mentioned a review by Richard Brown, M.D., of seven studies between 1982 and 1992 involving 566 patients. The studies reportedly indicated that opioids successfully treated chronic back pain, phantom limb pain, and *neuropathy,* while allowing some patients to return to work. Two of those studies reported fewer than 20% of patients were involved in "abusive behavior," while the other five reported no signs of addiction. (*Hippocrates,* November 1999, Vol. 13, No. 10).

Long acting opioids (**methadone, oxycodone, fentanyl**) are reported to have fewer cognitive side-effects, and provide better control of chronic pain. Also tolerance is believed to be less common than with the use of the shorter acting ones.

A concern of some practitioners is that the chronic use of opioids for pain will lead to life-threatening **respiratory depression.** (This is a decrease in the number of breaths or the depth of breathing.) Yet B. Eliot Cole, M.D., who instructs physicians in pain management through the AMA's Education for Physicians on End-of-Life Care (EPEC) program, maintains that patients who receive long-term opioid therapy have little risk in this regard. He says that once patients are up to a maintenance level, he would have to give them a massive increase to make respiration stop.

Gavril Pasternack, M.D., head of molecular neuropharmacology at Memorial Sloan-Kettering Cancer Center, says that there is **no ceiling** effect on opioids and that more pain relief will be provided with increasing administration.[78] He says that so long as dosage is brought

---

[78] Dr. Richard Payne, previously mentioned in the reference to the article in *Oncology News International* above, cites a study where chronic cancer pain patients were given either a dose of 225 mg of ketoprofen, a non-opioid analgesic previously discussed, or 5 to 10 mg of morphine intramuscularly. Mean pain relief was the same for both. When the ketoprofen was increased three-fold, there was no proportional degree of pain relief. However when the morphine was increased the patients experienced significant additional relief. The morphine doses at the increased level ranged up to a reported 35,000 mg (that's not a misprint). Dr. Payne observed that "there is a wide variability in the response to opioids, but there is no intrinsic ceiling."

up gradually, the respiratory system will become accustomed to the drugs and respiratory depression will not be a problem.

It is recognized that in some instances, opioid therapy alone may not provide sufficient analgesia for the treatment of neuropathic pain. Two recent studies seem to bear this out.

In the first, reported in *Doctor's Guide* (March 2, 2000), **epidural morphine** alone and a combination of clonidine HCL injection (Duraclon) and epidural morphine were administered to two groups of cancer patients. The clonidine/morphine combination provided significantly better analgesia than morphine alone (45 percent vs. 21 percent, respectively), according to the investigators. They also said the combination provided relief to 56 percent of patients with neuropathic pain versus 5 percent of those receiving just the morphine. (It should be pointed out that the study was conducted by clinicians at Roxane Laboratories, who developed Duraclon.)

The other was a randomized, placebo-controlled, double-blind trial with 12 volunteers in which the interaction of morphine and gabapentin was studied. The investigators found that the gabapentin "enhanced the acute analgesic effect of morphine."[79] (I suppose they could just as well have said the morphine enhanced gabapentin's effect!)

The most common adverse side effect of opioids is

[79] *Anesthesia and Analgesia* (2000 Jul; 91(1): 185–91).

constipation,[80] which is said to be best managed with a combination of laxatives and stool softeners, exercise, high-water/high-fiber diet, and avoidance of additional constipating medications (such as tricyclic antidepressants). These techniques, however, do not always work. A study which recognized this problem in situations where opioids are being administered long term, points to a different approach, at least in so far as methadone is concerned.

In a double-blind, randomized, placebo-controlled trial conducted between May 1997 and December 1998, **methylnaltrexone,** an **opioid receptor antagonist,**[81] was administered to 11 subjects and placebo to another 11, all who had methadone-induced constipation, to determine **laxation** (a nicer way to say bowel movement) response. The "oral-cecal transit times" (I didn't find that one in my medical dictionary but I figure it means how long from in to out) at baseline for subjects in the methylnaltrexone and placebo groups averaged 132.3 and 126.8 minutes, respectively. (Showing appropriate solicitude, the investigators apparently gave the good stuff to those who needed it most.) The average change for the methylnaltrexone-treated group was 37.2 minutes, which the investigators called "significantly greater" than the average change in

---

[80] For example, about 40% of patients on oral morphine are said to be constipated.

[81] The term "antagonist" refers generally, as here, to a chemical acting to reduce the physiological activity of another chemical substance. It is also often used to mean a chemical that opposes the action in the nervous system of a drug or a substance which occurs naturally in the body, by combining with and blocking its nervous receptor.

the placebo group—12.0 minutes. The investigators also said there was "no significant adverse effects" reported by the subjects during the study. (One can only guess at what they might have been.)[82]

2. Tramadol (Ultram)

Before leaving the subject of opioids, a "near opioid" should again be discussed. **Tramadol** (trade name **Ultram**) is considered an effective pain reliever for various purposes. Its mode of action resembles that of narcotics (in fact it is a synthetic analog of codeine). Tramadol is said, though, to have significantly less potential for abuse and addiction than most narcotics (even though both may occur). Also it reportedly does not depress respiration.

Toes and Soles discussed the 1998 study at Baylor College of Medicine in which 131 patients with diabetic neuropathy were treated with 210 mg of tramadol per day for six weeks, following which the investigators concluded that the drug was "significantly" more effective in treating neuropathic pain than placebo.

The same group of investigators did a follow-up study on 117 of the original 131 patients, assessing tramadol's

---

[82] I hope I have not offended anybody by my side remarks because I know constipation can cause serious distress, but I had to let go here. (No pun intended.) But really, I'm all for a little relief. To prove it, they've even (partially) named a herbal potion after me—"senna"—which is used for just this purpose. Read all about it in the article, "Managing Morphine-induced Constipation: a Controlled Comparison of an Ayurvedic Formulation and **Senna**," *Journal of Pain Symptom Management* (1998 Oct; 16(4): 240–44). Just kidding, of course (but the citation is correct).

long-term effectiveness.[83] In this investigation all 117 were placed on tramadol for six months. Pain intensity reports and pain relief scores were followed and tabulated. At the beginning of the extension, as the earlier study had indicated, those who had formerly been on placebo had "significantly higher mean pain intensity scores" and lower pain relief scores than those who had been on tramadol. At the end of the first 30 days of the extension in which all were on tramadol, pain *relief* scores had merged and were similar at the higher relief levels which had prevailed for the original tramadol group, and at the end of 90 days pain *intensity* scores had become similar at the lower levels for the original tramadol group. (Get it? In other words once those who had been on placebo began to take tramadol, they experienced the same benefits as those who were kept on tramadol all along.) The researchers drew what would seem to have been the appropriate conclusion: "Tramadol provides long-term relief of the pain of diabetic neuropathy."

Sindrup et al. performed an interesting study in 1999 where the object was to determine whether tramadol was effective in reducing **allodynia.**[84] (As indicated earlier, this is touch-evoked pain, or the perception of pain caused by usually nonpainful stimuli, such as touch or vibration.) The study was undertaken because, according to the investigators, it had been generally assumed by others that opioids—which tramadol resembles to some

---

[83] *Journal of Diabetes Complications* (2000 Mar-Apr; 14(2): 65–70).

[84] *Pain* (1999 Oct; 83(1): 85–90).

degree in respect to its action—relieved neuropathic pain less effectively than nociceptive pain. They also said it was widely believed that opioids did not have any effect on key characteristics of neuropathic pain such as allodynia. The study was randomized and double-blinded, and involved 45 patients of whom 34 remained in until the end. Dosages of slow-release tramadol tablets were titrated to between 200 and 400 mg daily to one group with the other receiving placebo. During the two treatment periods of 4 weeks duration, patients rated pain, *paresthesia* and touch-evoked pain by use of 0–10 point numeric rating scales. Mechanical allodynia was induced by stimulation with an electronic toothbrush and was rated at the end of each treatment period with a similar scale. At the conclusion of the trial, ratings for pain and *paresthesia* were significantly lower for the treatment group, as were ratings of allodynia. The investigators concluded that "tramadol appears to relieve both ongoing pain symptoms and the key neuropathic pain feature allodynia in polyneuropathy."[85]

When tramadol is prescribed, the dosage is often set at 50–100 mg every 4–6 hours, up to 400 mg per day.

---

[85] In interesting counterpoint to the study just discussed in which tramadol appeared to have been regarded as equivalent to opioids, the same investigators studied the opioid versus not-opioid ("monoaminergic," or neuro transmitting) actions or effects of tramadol. They concluded that "the opioid effect" of tramadol—or more properly of its opioid metabolite-MI—standing alone, may be of some importance for on-going relief of neuropathic pain but that, in general, relief of neuropathic pain seems to depend on both tramadol's opioid and on its non-opioid actions and effects in combination. *Clinical Pharmacology and Therapeutics* (1999 Dec; 66(6): 636–41). Capisce?

Chapter 3

Other Medical Therapies: Current Views

As in *Toes and Soles,* the subject of other medical therapies here concerns mainly **non-pharmacological** approaches to PN treatment, either **hematological** or **nerve-based**. Also, with respect to the former, the therapies are directed to specific **auto-immune conditions** such as **CIDP (chronic inflammatory demyelinating polyneuropathy)** and **(GBS) Guillain Barre syndrome.** These particular neuropathies typically involve **muscle weakness, paralysis** or **respiration problems,** as well as **burning pain**.

This chapter updates the information presented in *Toes and Soles*, with reports of new studies and new techniques.

Hematological

The principal therapies in this group, **plasmapheresis** (sometimes referred to as **plasma exchange**), **IVIg,** and **immunosuppressant medications,** were covered in the first book in some detail.

To quickly review, in plasmapheresis the **blood plasma**, which contains the **antibodies** believed to attack the myelin sheath, is **mechanically removed** from the blood with the red and white blood cells being returned together with other fluids.

IVIg is a high dose solution of proteins called **gamma globulins** which contain antibodies **providing immunity** against disease. These antibodies are thought to **block** the action of the antibodies causing the **myelin damage**. IVIg is administered intravenously.

Immunosuppressant medications are chemicals, usually **steroids**, which **suppress the immune system** and give the body an opportunity to **re-myelinate** damaged nerves.

As discussed in *Toes and Soles*, a study by neurologists at St. Elizabeth's Medical Center in Boston, found the positive response to the three therapies among patients treated for CIDP or GBS to be **approximately the same**—between 40 and 60%.[1] However, the investigators found that there was greater "**functional improvement**" among the patients who had been given plasmapheresis. More recent studies seem to suggest, though, a slight **shift in favor** of IVIg's perceived efficacy. Whether this is due to merely an incidental clustering of skewed results, or a more profound trend, must await the test of time. (I'm beginning to sound like a clinician, right?)

---

[1] *Neurology* (1997 Feb; 48(2): 321–28).

In the first study I found that followed the conclusion reached in Boston, Italian investigators at the University of Milan, in reviewing various "case series and trials," seemed to agree at least as to two modalities. They concluded from their reviews that "short term IVIg efficacy" is "comparable to that of plasma exchange" in the treatment of CIDP.[2]

German investigators were not called upon to make comparisons but in a study reported in early 1998, Berlin researchers stated, after reviewing various "experimental data and clinical trials," that "IVIg is a promising immunomodulary therapy that has been shown to be effective" in such diseases as GBS, CIDP, and **multifocal motor neuropathy** (**MMN**).[3] They noted that IVIg has few side effects, with a small risk of transmitting infectious agents.[4]

Later in 1998, on the other side of the world, Japanese investigators at the Department of Neurology in the Nagano Red Cross Hospital, studied eight patients with CIDP who went through anywhere from 4 to 51 plasmapheresis sessions and who were given **steroid** (**prednisone**) therapy as well. The investigators concluded that plasmapheresis administered with "concomitant steroid

---

[2] *Multiple Sclerosis* (1997 Apr; 3(2): 93–7).

[3] Multifocal motor neuropathy is similar to CIDP except that MMN patients commonly have asymmetric weakness of the distal (far) muscles, while in CIDP, proximal (near) symmetric weakness is more common. Patients with MMN are said to rarely have significant sensory symptoms, unlike CIDP.

[4] *Journal of the Neurological Sciences* (1998 Jan 8; 153(2): 203–14).

therapy is very useful for both short and long term treatment of CIDP patients."[5]

Another immunosuppressive agent, **cyclosporin A (CsA),** was retrospectively reviewed at the University of Sydney, Australia, in 19 patients with CIDP who had not responded to plasmapheresis, IVIg, or other immunosuppressive agents. The investigators concluded that CsA is "an efficacious and, with appropriate monitoring, safe therapy for patients with CIDP."[6]

As reported in October 1998, other Italian investigators (the lead investigator was the same as in the earlier Italian study) at the University of Milan, said simply that controlled trials demonstrated that IVIg, steroid treatments, and plasma exchange, are effective for CIDP.[7]

Clinicians at the Department of Neurology, Hospital of the University of Pennsylvania, shortly thereafter noted that plasma exchange had been shown effective in improving recovery time in GBS in several controlled trials during the 1980s but that IVIg therapy in the 90s had been demonstrated to be equally effective. They noted that IVIg offered advantages by being better tolerated in some patients and being easily administered without special equipment.[8]

As reported early the following year, Japanese investigators compared IVIg with **cyclophosphamide**, an-

---

[5] *Rinsho Shinkeigaku* (1998 Mar; 38(3): 208–12).
[6] *Muscle and Nerve* (1998 Apr; 21(4): 454–60).
[7] *Italian Journal of Neurological Science* (1998 Oct; 19(5): 261–69).
[8] *Neurology* (1998 Dec; 51(6 Suppl 5): S-15).

other immunosuppressant medication, in the treatment of MMN. They found that IVIg resulted in a superior outcome compared with the chemical, which they said sometimes caused serious adverse effects.[9]

Ten patients with MMN were treated with IVIg over a five day period at the Guy's King's and St. Thomas School of Medicine in London, as reported in July 1999. Four of the 10 showed a positive response to IVIg, with the best response occurring in two of them who presented with weakness but without severe muscle wasting. Three of the four continued to receive IVIg after the testing period with continued beneficial effect. The investigators concluded IVIg "should be considered" in patients with MMN.[10]

Again concerning multifocal motor neuropathy, nine patients in the Netherlands who had previously responded favorably to IVIg were treated with **interferon-beta 1a** (a chemical usually used for treating relapsing multiple sclerosis). Muscle strength and disability were evaluated for all of them. For six there was no treatment effect. In fact four deteriorated to such an extent that IVIg had to be restarted for them. Three reportedly showed an improvement with interferon-beta 1a that was more pronounced than with IVIg.[11]

A more recent study with 16 patients was conducted in the U.S. to determine the effect of IVIg on **neurological**

---

[9] *Rinsho Shinkeigaku* (1999 Jan; 39(1): 107–109).

[10] *Journal of Neurology, Neurosurgery and Psychiatry* (1999 Jul; 67(1): 15–19).

[11] *Neurology* (2000 Apr 11; 54(7): 1518–21).

function and **conduction block** in MMN.[12] They were assigned according to a randomized, cross-over design under double-blind conditions and given either IVIg or placebo (dextrose or saline) for five consecutive days. Patients were evaluated before and about 28 days after trial treatment for subjective functional improvement, neurological disability score, grip strength, distal and proximal compound muscle action potential amplitude, and conduction block. The subjective functional improvement with IVIg treatment was rated as "dramatic or very good" in nine patients, moderate in one, mild in one, and absent in five patients. Conduction block was reversed in five patients with IVIg. No improvements occurred in any of these respects with the placebo group.

In an editorial entitled "Easy to Start but Difficult to Stop," in the same issue in which the above study was reported, the authors stated that:

> IVIg is an effective but expensive treatment for patients with MMN. It is relatively easy to administer and the side effect profile is good. When patients with MMN improve after the initial IVIg course, it is very likely that maintenance treatment will be necessary. Because most patients and their physicians then wish to continue treatment, it is difficult to stop IVIg simply because of cost. Therefore, new studies should evaluate the effect of new, less-toxic immunomodulatory drugs that can be administered in conjunction with IVIg in order to reduce (or even replace) IVIg maintenance dosage and to further improve the clinical condition.[13]

---

[12] *Neurology* (2000; 55:1256–62).
[13] Ibid., 1246–47.

A recent review of 92 reports on the use of IVIg in neurological diseases in general compared it with other treatments.[14] Evidence was graded according to the design of the clinical trial, with the greatest weight being given to randomized, double-blind, controlled trials and the least to observational studies and case reports. For GBS and CIDP, studies suggested that IVIg and plasmapheresis were nearly equivalent in effectiveness, with neither superior to the other. Multifocal motor neuropathy had a good *initial* response to IVIg, but maintenance of response with continued treatment was found to be poor.

Another study looked at IVIg from a different point of view; rather than comparing it with other treatments for neurological diseases in general, this one considered *for which* neurological diseases it was most appropriate. Based on a synthesis of 92 studies, case reports and clinical observations, the following clinical recommendations were made by the investigators: it is *strongly* recommended for the treatment of GBS; *favorably* recommended for the treatment of CIDP and MMN; recommended as a *second resort* for the treatment of multiple sclerosis and myasthenia gravis; and recommended as a *last resort* for the treatment of polymyositis (inflammation of several muscles at once), inclusion-body myositis (muscular discomfort or pain from infection or an unknown cause), and intractable epilepsies.[15]

---

[14] *Journal Watch Neurology* (1 January 2000).

[15] *Canadian Journal of Neurological Sciences* (1999 May; 26(2): 139–52).

What do we take away from these studies? It seems to me, based on reported functional improvement and ease of administration versus side effects, that the investigators for the most part have tipped the scales to IVIg as the preferred treatment for CIDP, GBS, and multifocal motor neuropathy. The high cost of IVIg therapy, which was not a criterion in these studies, remains a practical problem of affordability for many, however. Obviously your doctor, based on knowledge of your situation, including tolerability of the various treatments, will have a significant contribution to make to the final decision if you suffer one of these syndromes.

Nerve-Based Treatments

1. Nerve Blocks

As described in *Toes and Soles*, a **nerve block** involves the injection of either a **local anesthetic** or a **neurolytic** (nerve destructive) agent into a peripheral nerve to decrease or eliminate nerve activity. A local anesthetic is often used to assess the likely effect of a more **permanent block**. Where a neurolytic agent is used the effect is to **destroy** many of the nerve fibers with which the agent comes into contact, thereby (hopefully) giving long-term relief from pain.

Most of the early studies on this procedure had reportedly shown it to be anywhere from 50 to 80% effective. I decided to go back and take a quick look at a few of them to see what the investigators had to say at the time they were performed, compared with current views. As you will see, the comments present a mixed picture as to their value.

In a 1981 investigation reported in the *British Medical Journal*, eight patients were studied in whom a lesion within the central nervous system had caused constant pain and **hyperpathia** (disagreeable or painful sensations in response to a normally innocuous stimulus such as a touch). Blockade was achieved by **stellate ganglion block** or intravenous infusion of **guanethidine**. The investigators reported that in almost every case the pain and hypersensitivity were reduced and in some cases completely eliminated.[16]

A group of German clinicians in 1987 noted that treatment of chronic pain through temporary or permanent nerve blocks had been "marked by great success." (They reported that in 792 blocks using neurolytic drugs, 96% were accomplished with ethyl alcohol and most of the rest with ammonium sulphate.)[17]

A 1989 randomized study compared the use of **phenol** and **cryogenic** (extremely low temperature) peripheral nerve **blocks** for 28 patients. The investigators reported that more patients in the phenol group received relief at 2, 12 and 24 week intervals than those in the cryogenic group. Overall, however, they found only 27% of patients received "significant relief," indicating to the investigators that "neurolytic blocks were not particularly effective." They added, though, that "*local* anesthetic

---

[16] *British Medical Journal* (Clin Res Ed 1981 Mar 28; 282(6269): 1026–28).

[17] *Regional Anaesthesia* (1987 Apr; 10(2): 55–58).

blocks produced significant but temporary pain relief [my emphasis]."[18]

A 1990 Swedish study involved 38 patients with neuralgia (acute pain radiating along the nerves) after peripheral nerve injury, who were treated with **local** anesthetic blocks. They all were said to have experienced relief of ongoing pain for 4 to 12 hours. There was a period of complete pain relief for 13 of the patients of 12 to 48 hours and of two to six days for another five.[19]

Another Swedish study six years later considered the **long-term** effects of nerve blockage. The cases of 45 patients with various pain symptoms were reviewed retrospectively. Only six were found to have experienced pain relief longer than a month. The researchers concluded from this that treatment with nerve block alone is "not very effective as a long-term treatment" for pain.[20]

Several more recent studies were found concerning the use of this procedure. One performed in 1998 involved 75 patients who were administered **butamben** (a local anesthetic) blocks, with 54 successfully treated. Mean duration for relief for 48 cancer patients was 12 weeks versus 10 weeks for six in the non-cancer group. Interestingly, there was a 75% decrease in opioid therapy for the cancer patients.[21]

A "critical review of the literature" was undertaken in

---

[18] *Journal of Pain Symptom Management* (1989 Jun; 4(2): 72–75).

[19] *Pain* (1990 Dec; 43(3): 287–97).

[20] *Journal of Pain Symptom Management* (1996 Mar; 11(3): 181–87).

[21] *Regional Anesthesia and Pain Medicine* (1998 Jul-Aug; 23(4): 395–401).

New Zealand at about the time of the last study. The researchers there found "little support for the widely-held view" that blocks reduced long-term neuropathic pain. They maintained that the literature supported the view that blocks were "only part of a balanced pain treatment strategy aimed at getting patients activated under cover of good analgesia and improved function."[22]

A similar study directed to a "review of the literature" was conducted at the University of New Mexico School of Medicine in 2000.[23] This one specifically covered the use of nerve blocks in the management of peripheral neuropathy, encompassing both local anesthetic and neurolytic procedures as well as **perineural** (into the nerve) **steroid injections**.

Stephen E. Abram, M.D., the investigator in the study, said that the local anesthetic blocks described in the literature seemed to have provided "useful **diagnostic information**" but tended to furnish only **temporary** therapeutic **benefits** for PN patients. He wrote that perineural steroids gave lasting relief for some, but that most studies indicated long-term relief was provided for only a minority of patients. He found from his review that peripheral neurolytic blocks seemed to be helpful to some patients with **mononeuropathies**, particularly where associated with cancer pain.

As noted in *Toes and Soles*, part of the problem in achieving long-term efficacy with the use of nerve blocks,

---

[22] *Regional Anesthesia and Pain Medicine* (1998 May-June; 23(3): 292–305).

[23] *Clinical Journal of Pain* (2000 Jun; 16(2 Suppl): S56–61).

where such is the goal, may be that nerves sometimes have the ability to regenerate themselves. Noting this risk, which can lead to pain recurrence as well as to other long-term complications, Dr. Abram said that relatively few physicians are willing to use peripheral neurolytic blocks for non-cancer pain.[24]

2. Direct Nerve Stimulation

Over the past thirty years various types of nerve stimulation techniques have been used to ease neuropathic pain.[25] It has been increasingly recognized that **electrical stimulation** of nerves for patients with peripheral neuropathy is not only effective in many cases but avoids the adverse side effects often involved with pharmacological agents.[26] Interesting and positive new developments have taken place in this area over the last few years. Some of them revolve around a technology/therapy called "**percutaneous** (through the skin) **electrical nerve stimulation**" or **PENS.**

---

[24] Dr. Abram referred to an earlier study which cited 17 lawsuits based on complications of neurolytic blocks, with all but one involving non-cancer patients.

[25] "The Future of Peripheral Nerve Neurostimulation," *Neurological Research* (2000 Apr; 22(3): 299–304); "Neuromodulation: Spinal Cord and Peripheral Nerve Stimulation," *Current Review of Pain* (2000; 4(5): 374–82). Authors of the latter report maintained that "Efficacy studies consistently show an overall 50% improvement in long-term pain control [using spinal cord and peripheral nerve stimulation] in patients who have failed conservative or other invasive modalities."

[26] *Southern Medical Journal* (1998 Oct; 91(10): 894–98).

(a) PENS

This procedure involves the insertion of very fine needles—usually 32 gauge, about the thickness of a human hair—into soft tissue or muscles. Electrical impulses are then delivered which stimulate peripheral nerves and promote the release of endorphins,[27] according to Dr. Paul White of Texas Southwestern Medical Center. He said that patients describe the feeling variously as sensations of "tapping, raindrops falling or a massage."

The procedure is similar in some respects to **electro-acupuncture** (see "Acupuncture" in Chapter 5) except that the probes are placed in areas where the physician has determined **nerve endings** are located. (Acupuncture, and variations thereof such as acupressure, involve the identification of channels of energy—qi—running through the body. These channels are called "meridians." Thin stainless steel needles are then placed at points along these meridians which may or may not relate to nerve ending points. Heat or electrical current is sometimes applied to the imbedded needles.)

According to some practitioners of PENS, patients may require 20 or more treatments. Based on patient responses, **adjustments** are often made to **electrical frequency** and **probe placement** during the treatment course.

Dr. White points out that the use of PENS reduces the

---

[27] As previously noted, endorphins are neurotransmitters produced by the brain that can have a powerful effect in reducing pain.

need for analgesic medications. In this regard he says the procedure is designed to complement, not eliminate, other pain management techniques. He also noted that it decreases the need for other more invasive procedures such as spinal cord stimulation (involving surgically placed implants, as explained later).

The earliest study I came across involving the use of PENS, however, was not directed to pain treatment. In a 1977 paper entitled "Electrical Stimulation for the Control of Pain," the use of the technique was considered "in predicting the **efficacy** of **implantable stimulators**," and according to the author, is meant to serve "the same function as diagnostic block."[28]

Later studies where PENS was used as a **therapy** were directed principally to cancer pain[29] and lower back pain.[30] The clinical study most often cited concerning the use of PENS with **peripheral neuropathy** took place in

---

[28] *Archives of Surgery* (1977 Jul; 112(7): 884–88).

[29] Study conclusion: "PENS therapy is a useful supplement to opioid analgesics for the management of pain secondary to bony metastasis in terminal cancer patients." *Clinical Journal of Pain* (1998 Dec; 14(4): 320–23).

[30] Study conclusion: "PENS was more effective than TENS [to be discussed] or exercise therapy in providing short-term pain relief and improved physical function in patients with long term LBP [lower back pain]." *JAMA* (1999 Sep 8; 282(10): 041–2).

Another study involving the use of PENS for lower back pain considered the effect of using different durations of electrical stimulation. The investigators "recommended that the duration be 30 minutes"—rather than the other two periods considered of 15 minutes and 45 minutes. *Anesthesiology* (1999 Dec; 91(6): 1622–27). Still another study concerning lower back pain evaluated the most appropriate frequencies of electrical stimulation to achieve optimal analgesia. Comparing alternations among 4 Hz, 15 Hz, 30Hz, and 100 Hz

2000 at the University of Texas Southwestern Medical Center at Dallas.[31] Fifty adult patients with Type 2 diabetes and peripheral neuropathy pain of more than six months involving the lower extremities, were divided into two groups. One received PENS with electrical stimulation of 15 and 30 Hz and the other sham (placebo) needles. The treatments were given over three weeks, 30 minutes three times a week.

At the conclusion of the study investigators found pain scores had been cut in half for the PENS group, with no change in the sham group. Also, improvement was noted in physical activity, sense of well-being, and the quality of sleep in the first group. Significantly, daily oral non-opioid analgesic requirements decreased by 49 and 14%, respectively, after active PENS and sham treatment.[32]

---

frequencies, the investigators concluded the 15 HZ alternating with the 30 Hz the best. [Authors query: Why is it that given three items in a range, the conclusion of medical investigators always seems to be to settle on the middle one. I think a meta analysis should be undertaken—by somebody else—to examine the validity of that observation, and then to delve into the psychological reasons of why that is so if my hypothesis is borne out. Just kidding, of course. But how about it? A cynic might say that the choice is frequently made before the study is instituted and that the two extremes are purposely set up to bracket the "correct" conclusion.)

[31] *Diabetes Care* (2000 Mar; 23(3): 365–70).

[32] In a study reported later in 2000, Dr. White's group studied the difference in results based on *where* the needles were placed in patients with **neck pain** and found a significantly greater reduction in pain, as well as increases in physical activity ability and quality of sleep, if they were inserted in the neck versus in the lower back. (They needed a study for that?) They also found the need for oral analgesic medications was decreased by an average of 37% for the neck-placement group versus 9% for the back group. *Anesthesia and Analgesia* (2000 Oct; 91(4): 949–54).

(b) TENS

PENS is similar to another therapy involving the introduction of an electric current to underlying nerves, known as "**trancutaneous electrical nerve stimulation**" or **TENS**. (This was extensively discussed in *Toes and Soles* together with yet another procedure called "METS," standing for "microcurrent electrical therapy stimulation.") With TENS, electrodes are placed **on the skin** near or at the location of the perceived pain. In contrast, because the PENS needles penetrate the skin, the electrical stimulus can be delivered closer to the nerve endings. (Proponents of PENS claim that this penetration also permits the needles to bypass the resistance of the cutaneous barrier.)

A study reported late in 1999 compared the efficacy of PENS with TENS in dealing with sciatica (pain along the course of a sciatic nerve in the back of the thigh). Sixty four patients whose sciatica was due to lumbar disc herniation were treated either with PENS, TENS, or sham PENS. Based on pain scores, both PENS (42%) and TENS (23%) were significantly more effective than sham (8%). By another analysis, PENS was found to be significantly more effective than TENS in improving physical activity and quality of sleep. Importantly, in the overall assessment, 73% of patients said that PENS was the most desirable modality, versus 21% for TENS and 6% for sham.[33]

---

[33] *Pain* (1999 Nov; 83(2): 193–99).

However, proponents of TENS haven't exactly been asleep at the switch in trying to energize the use of their technology (excuse the puns). A patient with "severe, painful diabetic neuropathy" who was not able to sleep because of her pain was given TENS treatment 20 minutes each day for 17 days. At the end of the period she reported she had no pain and could sleep through the night. The investigators concluded that "application of TENS to the skin of the lumbar area may be an effective treatment for the pain of diabetic neuropathy."[34]

In a shoot-out between TENS and acupuncture, both were said to have shown "significant improvements" in pain reduction.[35] The study involved 60 elderly patients with back pain of at least six months who were randomized between the two therapies for four weeks of treatment. The improvements were said to have "outlasted the treatment period," but, in less than a ringing endorsement, the investigators added that "this trial cannot exclude the possibility that both treatments are 'placebos.'"

A study of a device somewhat similar to a typical TENS unit was reported in *Muscle and Nerve*.[36] Results from a "**magnetic nerve stimulation**" (**MNS**) device, reportedly using a novel figure-8 magnetic coil, were compared with those obtained from conventional electric nerve stimulation (ENS) in patients with "disorders of the peripheral nervous system." Based on positive muscular responses, the investigators sweepingly said that

[34] *Physical Therapy* (1999 Aug: 79(8): 767–75).
[35] *Pain* (1999 Jul; 82(1): 9–13).
[36] *Muscle and Nerve* (1999 Jun; 22(6): 751–57).

"this new technique is a promising first step toward the ultimate goal of replacing ENS with MNS."

(c) ALTENS

A somewhat related procedure to TENS is **ALTENS**, or "**acupuncture-like transcutaneous electrical nerve stimulation**."[37] A review of six randomized, placebo-controlled trials with 288 participants was conducted in 2000 to determine the comparative efficacy of the two procedures in the treatment of patients with chronic low back pain.[38] The reviewers found the "overall odds ratio" for improvement in pain was 7.22 to 1 for ALTENS versus placebo, and TENS versus placebo, 1.52 to 1.

(d) H-wave Therapy

Another therapy similar to TENS involves the use of a so-called **H-wave machine** to provide electrical stimulation to nerves through probes placed on the body. The signals from these machines have a frequency range between 2 and 60Hz and a "biphasic exponentially decaying

---

[37] The nomenclature of these various nerve stimulation strategies gets a little confusing. The principal differences revolve around whether the current conductors are (a) inserted (needles-PENS) or implanted (electrodes—SCS), or (b) applied to the surface of the skin—TENS, ALTENS or HWT—the latter to be discussed next. You will also see references to broader characterizations such as ENS and MNS, as in the preceding section, or DENS, an acronym which some commentators use to discuss "direct electrical nerve stimulation." (Oh mama mia!)

[38] *Cochrane Database System Review* (2000; (2): CD 000210).

waveform."[39] According to one manufacturer, this emulates the natural waveform found in nerve signals in the body and therefore "enables greater and deeper penetration of a low frequency current, whilst [obviously an English manufacturer] using significantly less power than other machines." According to that company, the use of their H-wave machines is much safer, less painful and more effective than any other form of electrotherapy to date.

(The claim of superior efficacy was not borne out in a study comparing the analgesic effects of H-wave therapy [HWT] and TENS on pain thresholds of 48 "healthy human volunteers."[40] In the randomized trial, investigators administered either HWT at 2 Hz or 60 Hz, or TENS at 110 Hz,[41] or placebo. Though both HWT and TENS showed significant increases in mechanical pain threshold measurements [i.e., a lessened sensitivity to pain] versus placebo, neither was found to have demonstrated much advantage over the other. Diminished pain sensitivity [hypoalgesic] following the procedures did per-

---

[39] TENS has a frequency range of 1 to 250 Hz and pulse durations of 50 to 200 microseconds, while HWT has a fixed-pulse duration of 16 microseconds.

[40] *Archives of Physical Medicine and Rehabilitation* (1999 Sept, 80(9):1001–1004).

[41] As to the most effective TENS parameters, investigators in another study examined the application of the therapy to four groups of "healthy human subjects" at various pulse durations (50 microseconds and 200 microseconds) and frequencies (4 Hz and 110 Hz) and found that the combination of only one—110 Hz and 200 microseconds—achieved consistent benefits. *Archives of Physical Medicine and Rehabilitation* (1998 Sep; 79(9): 1051–58).

sist slightly longer in the group that had received HWT at 2 Hz.)

Another study involving 26 subjects with diabetic neuropathy compared the effectiveness of **H-wave therapy** and **amitriptyline**.[42] This was a placebo-controlled, randomized investigation in which all participants were prescribed 50 mg of amitriptyline over a 20 week period, with some of the subjects assigned to electrotherapy and some assigned to placebo. Of the 14 patients in the electrotherapy group, 12 (85%) experienced symptomatic improvement with five (36%) experiencing complete relief. Nine patients in the placebo group were able to complete the treatment phase but only one enjoyed complete relief (resulting from the amitriptyline alone); the remainder experienced some relief on average but less than in the electrotherapy group.

While the investigators said they were not certain what mechanism provided the relief for the electrotherapy group, they postulated that the treatment "affected the circulatory status and improved the oxygen tension in peripheral nerves." They concluded that this form of therapy could be combined with a pharmacological agent such as amitriptyline to "augment symptomatic relief" in those with diabetic neuropathy.

In a "self-reporting" study concerning the effects of H-wave therapy on neuropathic symptoms in diabetic patients (average age about 74 years and duration of diabetes about 16 years), questionnaires were mailed to

---

[42] *Diabetes Care* (1998 Aug; 21(8):1322–25).

people who had used HWT machines for about 1.7 years on average.[43] Patients were asked about their symptoms prior to and following machine use and to evaluate the effectiveness of electrotherapy. Of the 34 patients who returned the questionnaires and who had diabetes, 24 (70%) reported some relief in pain and discomfort. The reduction in pain for these 24 patients was calculated to be about 44%, or about 2.0 points on an analog scale of 0 to 10.

(e) Cortex and Spinal Cord Stimulation

Toes and Soles discussed **cortex** and **spinal cord stimulation** accomplished through the use of **implanted electrodes** into which a current is introduced.

In a recent study of 10 cases involving cortex stimulators in patients who had either post stroke pain, phantom limb pain or post-traumatic neuralgia and whose pain had failed to respond to conventional treatments, the investigators found long term benefit for five of them.[44] The investigators, though noting that cortex stimulation seemed "an effective analgesic intervention in some patients with chronic neuropathic pain," said it was "difficult if not impossible to predict those patients who may respond to treatment."

In an earlier study (not reported in *Toes and Soles*), spinal cord stimulation had been administered to 200 patients with pain of various etiologies, including diabetic

[43] *The Journal of Foot and Ankle Surgery* (1998 May-Jun; 37(3): 191–94).

[44] *Pain* (2000 Feb; 84(2–3): 431–37).

neuropathy.[45] Patients were followed later for periods of six months to 12 years. Forty two percent were found to have been able to control their pain by the use of spinal cord stimulation alone. Eleven percent needed occasional analgesic supplements. Pain associated with diabetic neuropathy, multiple sclerosis and sympathetic dystrophy "responded well," while phantom limb and paraplegic pain "responded poorly."

Three later studies affirmed the positive role that spinal cord stimulation can play in reducing **refractory pain** symptoms.[46] In the study reported in the *New England Journal of Medicine*, a comparison was made in treatment outcomes between two groups of patients, all with chronic reflex sympathetic dystrophy (a.k.a. complex regional pain syndrome). The 24 patients in the first group were given both spinal cord stimulation, with an implanted device, and physical therapy. The 12 patients in the second group received only physical therapy. The researchers found that pain improvement scores were "much higher" in the first group. Further, "health-related quality of life" scores were improved only in that group.

---

[45] *Axone* (11997 Jun; 18 (4): 71–73). The idea behind spinal cord stimulation is that, according to the "gate theory" of pain first propounded by Melzak and Wall (briefly discussed in Chapter 1), large diameter nerve fibers have the ability to "close the gate" at the spinal cord to the small-diameter nerve fibers which carry pain signals; the stimulation of these large fibers by a low voltage electrical current blocks or "gates out" the pain signals from reaching the cortex where pain is registered.

[46] *Archives of Medical Research* (2000 May 1; 31(3): 258–62); *Spine* (Aug 1; 25(15): 1886–92); *New England Journal of Medicine* (2000 Aug 31; 343(9): 618–24).

The researchers did note that six of the 24 patients in the first group had complications that required additional procedures, including removal of the implanted device from one.

As an indication of how a major health insurer views the "bona fides" of the procedure/therapies covered in this section, as well as exemplifying what an insurance company might cover, I thought you might be interested in the following. These are extractions from a Policy Bulletin on Electric Stimulation from Aetna U.S. Healthcare. (As stated , their Policy Bulletin applies to all fully insured Aetna U.S. Healthcare HMO, POS and PPO plans.)

As an inclusionary/exclusionary principal, Aetna considers whether the effectiveness of a particular procedure "has been established in the peer reviewed medical literature."

Covered is transcutaneous electrical nerve stimulation "when used as an adjunct or as an alternative to the use of drugs in the treatment of chronic, intractable pain." When TENS is used for that purpose, Aetna covers rental of the TENS unit for a one-month trial. After this one-month trial period, purchase of the TENS unit can be approved if it significantly alleviates pain and if the attending physician or physical therapist documents that the patient is likely to derive significant therapeutic benefit from continuous use of the unit over a long period of time.

The only coverage of percutaneous electrical nerve stimulation is for up to a 30-day period for the treatment of "chronic low back pain secondary to degenerative disc disease," when PENS is used as "part of a multimodality rehabilitation program that includes exercise." Peripheral neuropathy treatments apparently would not be covered.

H-wave stimulation is covered for patients who have "failed to adequately respond to conventional treatments of diabetic peripheral neuropathy."

Peripherally-implanted nerve stimulators are covered for treatment of "intractable neurogenic pain" when a number of criteria are met including "objective evidence of pathology (e.g., electromyography)" and that "a trial of transcutaneous stimulation was successful (resulting in at least a 50% reduction in pain)."

Chapter 4

More on Nutrient Supplementation

The bias among some in the medical profession against the use of **nutrient** or **dietary supplementation**[1] (the terms are interchangeable, at least as used here), and other alternative strategies for dealing with PN, was noted in *Toes and Soles.* A view not infrequently expressed, for example, is that because nutrient supplements do not undergo the same kind of testing as is required for new drug submissions to the FDA, their use should be restricted or perhaps even banned in some cases.[2] Those holding that view often contend there

---

[1] The Dietary Supplement Health and Education Act defines dietary supplements in general as products (other than tobacco) intended to supplement the diet that bears or contains one or more of the following dietary ingredients: a vitamin, mineral, amino acid, herb or other botanical.

[2] In his book, *World Without Cancer* (American Media 1997), G. Edward Griffin says that today's allopathic (conventional medicine-based) physicians should not be blamed if their practices are centered around the dispensing of drugs since medical schools have been preaching that approach for decades. He said that relates back to the beginning of the 20th century when John D. Rockefeller, Sr., gave

have been instances where apparently benign supplements, for example certain herbs, have caused dangerous side effects. However, when one looks at the reports of FDA-approved drugs being withdrawn from the market for safety reasons, sometimes after having produced devastating results, any overarching concern about the dangers of nutrient supplements *per se*—many of which have a long history of safe use—seems a bit ludicrous. (According to a recent CBS HealthWatch report, between 1993–98 the FDA received 2,600 reports of problems and 101 deaths linked to herbal supplements. Meanwhile, the report continues, *every year* 100,000 people die from problems associated with traditional drugs in the United States.)

This all, of course, is not to say that possibly adverse side effects of some supplements should be ignored. These side effects just shouldn't serve as a basis, in my opinion, for categorically denying the use of these substances because they haven't gone through the same battery of testing as have conventional medications.

Another view—which in the past had more validity than now—is that many supplements have been overhyped in their marketing. However, in the mid-90s, as discussed in *Toes and Soles,* comprehensive legislation was enacted and regulations adopted which significantly restrict advertising claims for dietary supplements. Now

---

enormous grants to medical schools with the stipulation that his representatives be placed on their boards. According to Griffin, these men then had a say in establishing curriculum that, because of Rockefeller's financial interests in the pharmaceutical industry, leaned heavily on drug therapy.

there are far fewer abuses by supplement manufacturers in making unsupportable claims. Those who flaunt these restrictions now face stiff penalties, including forced withdrawal of their products from the markets.

To further strengthen consumer protection, in March 1999, the Food and Drug Administration began requiring that labels list **all ingredients** of dietary supplements in order of quantity. Herbal products also have to specify the **part** of the **plant** used. Further, the labels must contain the **suggested "serving size"**—although I had never seen one that didn't—and information on nutrients "present in **significant levels.**"

Finally, some contend that in any event a well-balanced diet gives anyone all the nutrients they need. Studies, however, show just the opposite. Few Americans (let alone citizens of other countries who are behind us nutritionally) reach the RDA (recommended daily allowance) for most nutrients—modest goals indeed. The evidence seems quite clear that supplementation is important and can yield positive benefits for almost anyone.[3] If this is true with respect to ordinary, healthy human beings, how much more might this be true with those who have special needs—like us!

---

[3] An article in the prestigious and conservative *New England Journal of Medicine* (338:1060–61, 1998), maintains that people who take supplements are healthier than those who don't. Then again there are still, discouragingly, those, such as the medical director of one of the nation's leading diabetes centers, who dismissed supplements by simply saying if a specific *deficiency* cannot be found, "the vitamins will just go down the drain in your urine." ("Neuropathy Nerve Damage—An Update," Joslin Diabetes Center, 1999.)

This chapter contains **new information** from various studies, suggesting which nutrients can **especially** help us, and why. It will also briefly cover two **naturally derived substances,** not discussed in *Toes and Soles,* possibly having value for dealing with PN.

By the way and as mentioned in the Preface, there is no attempt here to rewrite *Toes and Soles;* that book should be referred to for basic information. Specifically, one should be certain to take the supplements mentioned there (again in consultation with your doctor) where significant evidence appears for their efficacy.

Vitamins

Although the information in *Toes and Soles* on the B complex and on vitamin C is not being repeated here, it needs to be understood that those vitamins are of **significant importance** to PNers and should be included in any supplement program. Attention should be paid particularly to taking the various family members of the **vitamin B complex** (including **biotin** and **inositol**) in a **balanced, combination** form, as set forth in *Toes and Soles.*

This section will cover important new data for PNers on three particularly critical vitamins. With respect to the first two (B1 and B12), the consequence of the **form** in which they are taken is highlighted, based on studies over the last several years.

1. Benfotamine

Stanley Mirsky was formerly the president of the New York affiliate of the American Diabetes Association. He claimed in his book, *Diabetes: Controlling it the Easy Way* (Random House 1998), that 80% of those with diabetic sensory neuropathy were improved after taking vitamin B1, or **thiamin.**

Toes and Soles discussed the usefulness of this nutrient for PNers. It did not distinguish, however, among the different forms of B1 in terms of relative effectiveness.

The one called **benfotamine** is a **lipid** soluble version which is more **bioavailable** (i.e., more available therapeutically to the body) than its **water** soluble counterparts, **thiamin hydrochloride** or **thiamin mononitrate.** (The result is that benfotamine is better at delivering thiamin into tissues where needed than the other forms.) The implication of this for us is that benfotamine should be even more beneficial in dealing with peripheral neuropathy than water soluble forms of B1. A number of studies, in fact, have borne this out.

First, an early investigation demonstrated the superior bioavailability of benfotamine among people in good health (remember, that's something we used to enjoy!).[4] Ten "healthy young men" were given oral administrations of either benfotamine or thiamin mononitrate. The researchers found that with a dose of only 40% of the for-

[4] *Annals of Nutrition and Metabolism (1991; 35(5): 292–96).*

mer compared with the latter, benfotamine provided "superior cellular efficacy."[5]

The classic and much cited study on the benefits of benfotamine for **treating neuropathy** was performed by H. Stracke et al.[6] In a double-blind, randomized, controlled study (those magical words which again makes peer acceptance possible), benfotamine, together with B6/B12, was administered over a period of 12 weeks to 24 patients with diabetic neuropathy. The researchers found a significant improvement in nerve conduction velocity and improvement in "vibration perception." The conclusion, stated with remarkable restraint based on the results, was that "the neurotropic benfotamine—vitamin B combination represents a starting point in the treatment of diabetic polyneuropathy." (You can't accuse these gentlemen of going out on a limb.)

The Stracke study was followed in 1997 by one in Bulgaria which compared the therapeutic efficacy of "**Milgamma**" tablets (50 mg benfotamine and .25 mg [sic] vitamin B12) with conventional vitamin B complex tablets.[7] Forty-five diabetes patients with peripheral neu-

---

[5] This conclusion was seconded in a paper presented at the 6th Symposium, "Vitamins and Additives in the Nutrition of Man and Animal," in 1997, where it was stated that a clinical study comparing the bioavailability characteristics of benfotamine and thiamin mononitrate administered to 20 dialysis patients, indicated a "considerably higher relative bioavailability" in the former B1 form. (No other details were given.)

[6] *Experimental and Clinical Endocrinology and Diabetes* (1996; 104(4): 311–16).

[7] *Folia Medica* (1997; 39(4): 5–10).

ropathy were divided into two groups and received the different treatments over a three-month period. At the end of the study the investigators said that "statistically significant relief of both background and peak neuropathic pain was achieved in all of the Milgamma-treated patients and vibration perception thresholds dramatically improved," while "symptom improvement was insignificant" among those on the conventional B complex regimen. With much greater enthusiasm than the Stracke crew, they proclaimed the Milgamma tablets "an indispensble element in the therapeutic regimen of patients with painful diabetic neuropathy."

A Russian study in 1998 also considered a Milgamma preparation—this one containing 100 mg of benfotamine and 100 mg of pyridoxine or vitamin B6—for the treatment of diabetic polyneuropathy. The treatment was administered to 14 patients three times a day for 6 weeks. At the end of the period the investigators said that pain scores were reduced from 8.2 to 2.3 (on a scale of 10), and that indices of vibratory sensitivity had improved significantly. They said there was an amelioration of the neuropathic condition in 93% of the cases.[8] A similar conclusion was reached at about the same time back in the United States where the **bioequivalence** (i.e., the degree to which the same bioavailability and physiological effects are provided) of three thiamin preparations were compared using seven volunteers with polyneuropathies. The researchers said that, "From our results it can be

[8] *Zh Nevrol Psikhiatr Im S S Korsakova* (1998; 98(9): 30–32).

concluded that oral administration of benfotamine is best suitable for therapeutical purposes owing to its excellent absorption characteristics."[9]

Benfotamine was once more pitted against a vitamin B combination (B6 and B12 in this case) in a placebo-controlled, double-blind study of 84 patients with "severe symptoms of alcoholic polyneuropathy."[10] The study was conducted over an eight-week period in Glessen, Germany, in 1998. Investigators said that "benfotamine led to significant improvement of alcoholic polyneuropathy."[11]

In 1999, Hungarian investigators considered the effects of different doses of benfotamine for patients with painful diabetic neuropathy. Thirty six patients were divided into three groups, the highest dosage group receiving 320 mg a day and the lowest, 150 mg daily. Five different parameters of neuropathy were assessed. The principal investigator, Dr. G. Winkler, and his associates found at the end of the study that although an overall beneficial therapeutic effect was observed in all three groups, the greatest change concerning neuropathic symptoms occurred among those receiving the highest dosage of benfotamine.[12]

---

[9] *International Journal of Clinical Pharmacology and Therapeutics* (1998 Apr; 36(4): 216–21).

[10] *Alcohol and Alcoholism* (1998 Nov-Dec; 33(6): 631–38).

[11] A study entitled "Alcohol and the Peripheral Nervous System," also makes the point that alcoholic polyneuropathy results from "inadequate nutrition, mainly deficiency of thiamin and other B vitamins." No distinction was made among the various forms of thiamin. (*Ther Umsch,* 2000 Apr; 57(4): 196–99).

[12] *Arzneimittelforschung* (1999 Mar; 49(3): 220–24).

Dr. H. Stracke at the University of Giessen in Germany, who was the lead investigator in the 1996 study previously mentioned, said in a an interview published in "The Experts Speak," that an "initial dose of 3 x 100 mg of benfotamine daily for two to three weeks followed by a dose of 1 to 2 x 100 mg," would be appropriate in dealing with diabetic neuropathy. He added that "the high lipid solubility [of benfotamine] leads to a better resorption [a process of breaking down and assimilation in the body] and thereby proves a higher tissue compatibility."[13]

It seems clear that for PNers, benfotamine is the form in which the important nutrient, vitamin B1, should be taken. Based on the foregoing information, a daily intake of 200–300 mg would seem generally sufficient for therapeutic purposes.

2. Vitamin B12

Vitamin B12 is the name for a group of biological compounds essential to the body known as **cobalamins.** The most common form is called **cyanocobalamin,** the more neurologically active **methylcobalamin,** or **methyl B12.**

Investigators have linked many central and peripheral neurological disorders to a deficiency in methyl B12. (See, e.g., "Methylcobalamin: A Potential Breakthrough in

[13] *Experimental and Clinical Endocrinology and Metabolism* (1996; 104: 311–16).

Neurological Disease," HealthWatch, Winter 1999.) The reverse also has proven true, with significant neurological benefits demonstrated when methylcobalamin is made available to the body in adequate amounts.

Our bodies actually produce a small amount of this substance in the liver. However, much larger amounts of methylcobalamin are said to be required to correct neurological defects and also to neutralize a highly toxic substance produced in the body called **homocysteine.** This **amino acid** is linked to heart disease, stroke and other problems.[14]

Homocysteine tends to accumulate in the body when methyl 12 becomes deficient. (As will be explained later, measuring this accumulation is one way of determining whether the body is sufficiently and efficiently supplied with B12—too much homocysteine is definitely a problem from a general health standpoint!) If adequate quantities of methyl 12 and its synergistic cousin, **folic acid** or **folate,** are present, the body is then able to recycle the homocysteine to **methionine.** This substance in turn

[14] Studies released in February 2001, at a meeting of the American Stroke Association in Ft. Lauderdale, Florida, strengthened the case that elevated levels of homocysteine can lead to strokes. Dr. Peter J. Kelly of Massachusetts General Hospital in Boston, and his team, combined the results of 14 studies involving more than 11,000 patients. Together, they suggested that people with high levels of homocysteine have a 75 percent greater risk of stroke than do those with average levels. The analysis also showed that people who suffer strokes have average homocysteine levels that are 18 percent higher than those who do not. (No one knows precisely what the ideal homocysteine level is. However, doctors estimate that one-quarter of the U.S. population has clearly elevated levels.)

is further metabolized into the amino acid S-adenosylmethionine or **SAMe,** which was discussed in *Toes and Soles*.

The importance of SAMe is that it is used by the body in a **methylation** process which helps, among other things, to **regulate neurotransmitters**—mentioned before as chemical substances in nerve cells which relay pain messages to the brain.[15] In a supplement form, SAMe is sometimes used as an antidepressant, or for osteoarthritis.[16]

A good deal of the work involving methylcobalamin has been done in Japan, the only country where it could be fairly easily obtained (but with a prescription required) before 1998. Investigators there were reported in 1987 to have found that introducing a high concentration of methylcobalamin into **spinal fluid** was both highly effective and safe for treating the symptoms of diabetic neuropathy.[17]

A 1994 study went a step further and studied **nerve regeneration** in rats from ultra-high doses of methyl B12. The researchers concluded that the administration of 500 micrograms/kg daily resulted in a significant **en-**

---

[15] In a 1998 article in the *Journal of Neurological Neuro-Psychiatry,* there is a discussion of the underlying mechanisms and causes of neuropathy, and the role of oxidation on the methyl transfer cycle which causes a deficiency of SAMe. This report indicates that SAMe supplementation may be helpful in the treatment of neuropathy.

[16] I apologize if the technical stuff here seems a bit much but I think some understanding of how these substances interact in the body helps with an appreciation of their significance to our health.

[17] *Clinical Therapy* (1987; 9 (2): 183–92).

hancement in **nerve fiber density.**[18] (The typical human equivalent would be about 40 mg!) Their conclusion was that very high doses of methyl B12 could be helpful in treating peripheral neuropathies.[19]

A 1999 investigation examined the effect of methylcobalamin given **intravenously.** Nine chronic hemodialysis patients with diabetic neuropathy were administered 500 mcg injections three times a week for six months. The investigators found that at the end of that period the patients' pain and *paresthesia* had lessened and that **sensory nerve conduction velocities** had shown significant improvement.[20]

Injecting vitamin B12 **intramuscularly,** in either the methylcobalamin or cyanocobalamin form, has been the preferred method of administration for years for this nutrient. (B12 is used supplementarily for a variety of health reasons: for example cardiovascular problems, Alzheimer's disease, chronic fatigue syndrome, and sleep disorders.[21]) The belief has been that injections enhance absorption by the body more readily and provide speedy and direct availability.

---

[18] This was echoed in the *HealthWatch* article previously cited: "[H]igh doses of methylcobalamin are needed to regenerate neurons as well as the myelin sheath that protects nerve axons and peripheral nerves."

[19] *Journal of Neurological* Science (1994 April; 122(20): 140–43).

[20] *Internal Medicine* (1999 June; 38(6): 472–75).

[21] The level of B12 decreases with age, and age-related deficiencies are associated with such impairments as hearing and memory loss. According to one researcher, "Vitamin B12 deficiency is estimated to affect 10–15% of people over the age of 60." *Annual Review of Nutrition* (1999; 19: 357–77).

Recently, however, it has been argued that the **sublingual** (under the tongue) manner of taking this vitamin is just as effective as injections.[22] At the 28th World Congress of Hematology it was reported (Reuters, August 30, 2000) that Israeli investigators tested 18 patients with B12 deficiency. They found blood levels of B12 had increased in all patients to normal after only a few days following the sublingual ingestion of 1000 mcg of the vitamin twice a day. No side effects were reported.

A monograph in the *Alternative Medicine Review* maintained that there is no therapeutic advantage in any particular method: **orally, intramuscularly,** or **intravenously.**[23] (No mention or distinction was made between the usual oral method of taking a pill with water, or placing it under your tongue.)

A 1992 study concluded that **oral** administration of 500 mcg of methylcobalamin three times daily for three months, resulted in subjective improvement in burning sensations, numbness, loss of sensation, and muscle cramps. There was no indication whether or not the administration was sublingual.[24]

Some of the more recent studies concerning methylcobalamin have involved dosages as high as 25–60 mg

---

[22] This method permits the rapid absorption of substances directly into the blood stream rather than through the digestive tract as is true with the usual pill-with-water routine. Sublingual absorption avoids exposure to the dilutive effect of the gastric system and liver, resulting in a quicker and more efficient delivery.

[23] (1998 Dec; 3(6)).

[24] *Clinical Neurology and Neurosurgery* (1992; 94: 105–11).

per day for adult humans. (Incidentally, the RDA is 2 *mcg.*) The *Alternative Medicine Review* monograph cited above maintains the appropriate dosage for "clinical effect" is 1500–6000 mcg (1.5 to 6 mg) daily. The author argues that there is no therapeutic advantage in exceeding this level. The *Cecil Textbook of Medicine* (21st Ed., 2000, W. B. Saunders Company), states that 1000 to 2000 mcg (1 to 2 mg) daily is the "treatment of choice for most patients." The author also says that hematological and neurological responses are the same whether oral or parenteral (injected) administration is used.

The 1999 *HealthWatch* article previously mentioned suggests that PNers taking alpha-lipoic acid should **also take** at least 5 *mg* of sublingual methylcobalamin a day to make sure that the ALA would be bioavailable to the peripheral nerves. (In passing, the article made the point that since methylcobalamin is not a drug which anyone could have patented, there is no economic incentive to conduct costly clinical studies concerning it. This was the same point made concerning nutrients generally in *Toes and Soles.*)

Since, where a deficiency has been established, it may have taken a long time for the body's natural stores of B12 to become depleted, it may similarly take some while for restoration to be achieved. Dr. Lark Lands, a noted nutrition expert who advocates that regular doses of B12 be taken in the form of **injections** or **nasal gel,** says that it can take two to eight weeks (at least for AIDS patients) to return to normal B12 status if the deficiency is severe. She also warns in her upcoming book, *Positively Well: Liv-*

ing with HIV as a Chronic, Manageable, Survivable Disease (portions of which she has generously shared with me), that it is critical to replace depleted B12 as soon as possible; she points out that in the most advanced stage of B12 deficiency, any damage caused may not be reversible.

(Dr. Lands mentions a study by Dr. Martin David, Division of Geriatric Medicine, West Penn Hospital in Pittsburgh, where he found a very strong correlation between the duration of B12 "deficiency-induced cognitive symptoms" in the elderly and response to therapy with B12 injections. The best cognitive responses came from those who had been experiencing problems for less than six months. For those who had symptoms from six months to a year there was still a "fairly good response." He said that for those whose symptoms had lasted longer, even substantial supplementation with B12 did not make for improvement.)

There seems to be some confusion concerning appropriate **testing** for B12 deficiency. Typically many doctors have relied on simply measuring **serum (blood)** levels. The problem with this approach is that it does not reveal whether the B12 present in the blood is **available** to and is being properly used by the body, or if "**malabsorption**" is occurring.[25] More sophisticated tests, measuring the presence of elevated **methylmalonic acid (MMA)**

---

[25] Malabsorption can result from the lack of "intrinsic factor," a binding protein produced by cells within the stomach and required for the proper absorption of vitamin B12.

and **homocysteine (HCY)** levels—taken together—are considered better markers and more suggestive of the need for B12 supplementation.[26]

HCY levels are checked in a **blood test** and MMA in a **urine test.** If one or both indicate these levels are **too greatly elevated,** it may be tentatively assumed that the body is not well supplied with **available** B12. However, whether in fact the test results indicate a true B12 deficiency can only finally be determined after the fact by **re-testing** following the administration of B12 supplements, to see if there was an improvement (i.e., lowering) of HCY and MMA levels.

A personal view: based on the information I have seen, I am opting as a PNer to take 1000 mcg of methylcobalamin sublingually on a daily basis (together both with folate, a co-factor which recycles toxic homocysteine, and very importantly, with a B complex supplement), and not spend money on deficiency tests. Vitamin B12 is well tolerated, is not that expensive, and based at least on the suggestion of existing evidence, seems to provide neurological benefits whether or not there is a proven deficiency.

3. Vitamin E

This nutrient continues to draw interest as a major **scavenger** of **free radicals** in the body—those molec-

---

[26] See, e.g., the excellent article, "Laboratory Diagnosis of Vitamin B12 and Folate Deficiency," Snow, *Archives of Internal Medicine,* Vol. 159, June 28, 1999.

ular fragments which cause cell damage in various organs. Dr. William Haynes, in an article, "The 'Renaissance' of Vitamin E" (May 1998), writes about vitamin E's excellent **antioxidant** defenses against these free radicals, and points out its **protective effect** against such neurological diseases as Parkinson's and peripheral neuropathy.[27]

A study reported in the journal, *Metabolism,* tested the effects of this vitamin on oxidative stress and free radical damage in Type 2 diabetic patients. The investigators found that improving glycemic levels (i.e., lowering blood sugar levels) with dietary changes and drugs lowered oxidative stress somewhat, but when these patients were supplemented with vitamin E for four weeks, oxidative stress and free radical damage were further reduced, "almost to the level of healthy people."[28]

Earlier clinical studies demonstrated that low levels of vitamin E may lead to peripheral neuropathy.[29] The reverse was shown by a fairly recent double-blind, randomized, placebo-controlled study of 21 subjects with diabetic neuropathy performed in Ankara, Turkey. The investigators found that nerve conduction had been improved

---

[27] Article appears at *http://www.princetonol.com/family/columns/vitamin.html*. Dr. M. G. Traber, Associate Professor of Nutrition at The Linus Pauling Institute, argues, however, that although vitamin E (particularly in its alpha-tocopherol form, as discussed in *Toes and Soles*), is an excellent antioxidant, its greater importance lies in its regulation of "biological activities" such as metabolism.

[28] *Metabolism* (2000; 49: 160–62).

[29] See, e.g., *New England Journal of Medicine* (1987 Jul 30; 317(5): 262–65).

significantly by the administration of 900 mg (sic—query whether 900 IU was meant, and on what frequency basis) of vitamin E over a six month period.[30]

Investigators in a Dutch study where "high doses" of vitamin E were given to rats in which diabetic neuropathy had been induced, indicated "nerve dysfunction had been prevented by 50%."[31]

A Korean study (see, researchers all over the world are working on answers for us!) concluded that vitamin E-deficient neuropathy is reversible after four months of therapy with water-soluble vitamin E (there was no indication of the dosage used).[32]

As noted in *Toes and Soles,* many practitioners suggest vitamin E be taken in doses of 400–800 IUs daily. (A study of high doses in the treatment of neurological disorders in the elderly concluded that oral intakes of up to 2000 IUs daily was relatively safe for periods of up to two years. The investigators went on to say that "the safety and efficacy of supplemental vitamin E" over longer periods "had not been adequately explored.")[33]

An interesting investigation in Italy indicated the administration of vitamin E to children before the age of three could prevent or reverse neuropathies that might otherwise result from certain liver diseases.[34]

---

[30] *Diabetes Care* (1998 Nov; 21(11):1915–18).

[31] *European Journal of Pharmacology* (1999 Jul 9; 376(3): 217–22).

[32] *Archives of Physical and Medical Rehabilitation* (1999 Aug; 80(8): 964–67).

[33] *American Journal of Clinical Nutrition* (1999 Nov; 70(5): 793–801).

[34] *Acta Vitaminologica Et Enzymologica* (1985, 7 Suppl 33–43).

Minerals

These **inorganic nutrients** are involved in many biochemical processes supporting life. *Toes and Soles* identified and discussed four that are considered especially helpful in dealing with peripheral neuropathy: chromium, magnesium, selenium and zinc. The proper balance of these trace nutrients is especially important. This section deals with **new information** concerning all of them as well as a mineral not discussed in *Toes and Soles:* lithium.

1. Chromium

There is new evidence concerning the benefits of an adequate **chromium** supply for PNers, particularly for those with diabetic neuropathies, although some would dispute the necessity of **supplemental** amounts.

The new *Merck Manual of Diagnosis and Therapy* (17th Ed., Section 1, Chapter 4), reports a study of four patients with glucose intolerance and peripheral neuropathy. Three responded positively with doses of 150 to 250 mcg of **trivalent chromium,** with both a reduction in PN and an increase in glucose tolerance.

Diabetes Metabolism refers to a study in which a patient with "severe neuropathy and glucose intolerance," had been on "total parenteral [by injection] nutrition," at the time receiving currently recommended levels of chromium. The neuropathy and glucose intolerance reportedly were *reversed* by additional chromium supplementation.[35]

A study in the *Journal of the American College of Nutrition* concluded that although 200 mcg of chromium daily was adequate for those who are mildly glucose intolerant, people with "more overt impairments" require higher dosages.[36] Specifically, a daily intake of 8 mcg per kg body weight was mentioned. This would be equal to about 544 mcg for a person weighing 150 pounds.

There are still some who question—or at least need more convincing of—dietary supplementation of chromium being necessary for those with diabetes. For example at a workshop held by the Office of Dietary Supplements at the National Institutes of Health in November 1999, it was said:

> The overriding question left to the committee was what is the best way to derive further information to determine whether a deficient chromium status plays a role in the incidence of diabetes in this country. Most perplexing is the fact that we do not yet have a good measure of chromium status, we cannot measure or assess deficiency in people, and we have not developed satisfactory animal models that can be extrapolated to humans. Hence, it becomes evident that the development of appropriate and sensitive biomarkers and outcomes measures are pivotal prior to initiation of formal clinical in-

---

[35] (2000 Feb; 26(1): 22–27).

[36] *Journal of the American College of Nutrition* (1998 Dec; 17(6): 548–55).

tervention studies. *It is clear that, for the general public, current data do not warrant routine use of chromium supplements, whose risk-benefit function has not yet been adequately characterized.*

Incidentally, the recommendations reported in *Toes and Soles,* for those who have decided to use chromium in supplemental form, were in the range of 200 to 400 mcg daily. (Keep in mind we are talking about *micrograms,* not *milligrams* as with magnesium supplements. The former is 1/1000th of the latter.)

2. Magnesium

Magnesium is one of the minerals said to be necessary in proper amounts to enhance **nerve conduction** as well as for **other biochemical processes.** This mineral may be especially important for those with diabetes and diabetic neuropathy.[37] A recent paper reviewed a study of 35,988 older women who were initially free of diabetes. Of these, 1141 developed Type 2 diabetes within six years. The study determined that although dietary fiber intake led to the lowest chance to contract diabetes, the strongest **protective effect** was observed for magnesium consumption. Women who had consumed 332 mg of magnesium daily cut their risk of developing diabetes in half compared with women who consumed less than

---

[37] Dr. Lark Lands in her upcoming book points out that, in HIV patients, magnesium can be lost from their bodies as a result of infections and that any additional infections can greatly increase the likelihood of a magnesium deficiency.

242 mg daily.[38] (*Toes and Soles* noted that various doctors recommended adding 200 to 400 mg of magnesium daily as a supplement.)

3. Selenium and Zinc

A December 1998 study pointed out how **selenium** and **zinc** (as well as copper) are involved in the destruction of free radicals through "cascading enzyme systems."[39] The authors of the study said that the efficient **removal** of these **free radicals** maintains the integrity of membranes, reduces the risk of cancer, and slows the aging process. A point they made which was particularly interesting to me was the fact that *excessive intake* of these trace elements can lead to a number of problems, including neuropathy. Thus we must be careful not to "over-dose" when we take supplements duplicating trace minerals we may be getting in other ways, such as in a multi-purpose vitamin. (*Toes and Soles* set forth the total amounts of these minerals that various practitioners recommend for therapeutic purposes.)

The authors of the preceding study said it was important to differentiate whether the trace element **deficiency** (which was the focus of *Toes and Soles*), or the trace element **toxicity** (i.e., resulting from excessive intake), is the primary cause of the disorder (e.g., neuropathy). They point out, however, that these aspects may be

---

[38] *American Journal of Clinical Nutrition* (2000 Apr; 71(4): 921–30).

[39] *Clin Lab Med* (1998; 18(4): 673–85).

secondary to other factors (e.g., such as vitamin 12 deficiency, alcoholism, etc.). The authors maintain that only successful treatment of the **primary cause** will lead to complete recovery.

4. Lithium

In reviewing studies concerning mineral supplementation and its effects on peripheral neuropathy, I came across an interesting study in Japan in 2000 performed at the Osaka University Medical School. Clinicians there tested the effects of **lithium** on the symptoms of rats that had been experimentally subjected to peripheral neuropathy. (Lithium, as you may know, is usually administered to counteract acute manic episodes in patients with bipolar affective disorders. Also, maintenance therapy with the substance has been found useful in preventing or diminishing the frequency of subsequent relapses.)

The clinicians found PN symptoms reduced when they used **intrathecal** injections (injections administered under the membranes covering the brain or spinal cord) of lithium. Noting that this alkali metal already had found widespread clinical application, they said their results "suggested that its therapeutic utility may be extended to include treatment of neuropathic pain symptoms resulting from peripheral nerve injury."[40]

---

[40] *Pain* (2000 Mar; 85(1–2): 59-64). Not a bad translation of mine, don't you agree, considering I had only spent a few weeks in Tokyo after the Korean Conflict? Well, actually, I thought it would be better to rely on the multi-lingual editors at the journal *Pain* to extract the full meaning of the Osakans. I am sure you feel better about my doing that, too.

Curiously, other studies I found where lithium was mentioned in connection with peripheral neuropathy concerned its toxic effects and its propensity to *induce* PN.[41] That reminds one a little of vitamin B6 and its value, in appropriate amounts, as an aid with PN, as opposed to the dangers of its causing peripheral neuropathy if too much is taken.

Other Important Supplements

1. Essential Fatty Acids

Many people coming across the term "fatty acids" for the first time think they sound like something that should be definitely avoided. After all, we've been taught "fat" is not good for us—at least too much of it—and acids—well, they're better left in the laboratory. Of course the word "essential" does tend to put a different spin on it.

Toes and Soles discussed in brief the role of **essential fatty acids** or **EFAs,** in dealing with peripheral neuropathy. To start with, these are **polyunsaturated lipids,** not the saturated kinds of fats found in many animal products.

EFAs are components of **cell membranes** the body needs but cannot manufacture itself. Diets rich in polyunsaturated fats such as EFAs increase the fluidity

---

[41] See, e.g., "Lithium and its Effects on the Endocrine System, Bones and Peripheral Nerves," *Fortschr Neurol Psychiatr* (1995 Apr; 63(4):149–61).

of these membranes. On the other hand diets high in saturated fats tend to lead to rigid and unhealthy cell membranes.

EFAs are also precursors of **prostaglandins.** These latter substances are **hormones** which facilitate many processes such as energy production, the transfer of oxygen into the bloodstream and the manufacture of hemoglobin. In addition to transporting oxygen, their particular importance to us lies in their assistance in the transmission of nerve impulses and possibly in the enhancement of nerve regeneration.

There are two main EFA groups: **omega-3** and **omega-6** fatty acids. The terms refer to their differing chemical structures. Omega-3s are found in **cold water fish** such as sardines, herring, mackerel, salmon, and halibut, as well as **flaxseed oil.** (Non-fish eaters can also try marine plants such as seaweed supplied as **microalgae supplements.**)[42] Omega-6s are constituents of many vegetable oils such as **borage seed,** and **black currant,** as well as **evening primrose oil.**

Toes and Soles discussed the neuropathic benefits of **gamma linolenic acid (GLA).** This is a specific omega-6 fatty acid manufactured in the body by **linoleic**

[42] Artemis Simopolous, M.D., head of the Center for Genetics, Nutrition and Health in Washington D.C., points out that another plant, purslane, is not only rich in omega-3s but also contains vitamins E and C as well as beta-carotene and glutathione—all valuable for PNers, as discussed in *Toes and Soles.* Purslane can be eaten cooked like spinach, or used fresh in salads.

acid, another omega-6. Various foods actually contain small amounts of GLA, and the body produces the fatty acid on its own from a number of dietary fats.[43]

An investigation was described in *Toes and Soles* where a group of diabetic patients with neuropathy took 480 mg of GLA daily and were reported to have experienced a gradual **reversal** of **nerve damage** as a result of the re-building of the myelin sheath.

A recent study involving the use of GLA for diabetic neuropathy treatment in rats, found that this omega-6 was useful in **preventing** a **deficit** in **nerve conduction velocity** (NCV)—a test and marker for peripheral neuropathy.[44] Also the June 2000 issue of the German journal, *Fortschritte der Neurologie-Psychiatrie,*[45] reported that "evening primrose oil, containing gamma-linolenic acid, might improve nerve conduction velocities, temperature perception, muscle strength, tendon reflexes and sensory function."

Another study I came across in an Internet "bio FAQ"

---

[43] Evening primrose oil offers a concentrated source, with 7 to 10% of its fatty acids available in the form of GLA. However, borage oil contains even more GLA (20 to 26%), and black currant oil offers 14 to 19%. The effectiveness and safety of the latter two have not been as intensively examined as evening primrose oil. Nonetheless, some people prefer borage and black currant oils because they require a lower dose (at less total cost) for the same amount of GLA.

[44] *American Journal of Clinical Nutrition* (2000 Jan; 71(1 Suppl): 386S-92S). NCV is a measure of how fast electricity flows through a nerve. It is related to the diameter of the nerve and, sometimes, to the degree of its myelination (the presence of a myelin sheath on the axon).

[45] (2000 Jun; 68 (6): 278–88).

format also suggested that patients with *existing* neuropathies could experience improvement with GLA supplementation. Additionally, this study maintained that any one with diabetes might consider supplementing with borage oil—just mentioned as another omega-6 source—as a *preventive measure* against neuropathy. Two grams of borage oil daily was the recommended amount.[46] (Dr. Lark Lands, in her upcoming book, *Positively Well: Living with HIV as a Chronic, Manageable, Survivable Disease,* says that at least two borage oil capsules with 240 mg of GLA in each, taken on a daily basis, might be useful in dealing with neuropathy.)

Incidentally *Toes and Soles* reported an investigation concerning the **synergistic effect** of combining GLA and alpha-lipoic acid in the treatment of diabetic neuropathy.[47] This work was affirmed in a later study reported in the same journal. The conclusion reached was that alpha-lipoic acid by itself did not improve nerve conduction velocity—as just indicated, a marker of peripheral neuropathy—but a **conjugate** (a chemical compound formed by the union of compounds) of the two did so.[48] A study reported in *Diabetes Research and Clinical Practice,*

---

[46] The study, although claimed to be backed by scientists linked to the University of Saskatchewan, was presented at a commercial web site (www.bioriginal.com) where nutrients are sold. Bias thus obviously must be considered. However the overall article was an excellent, in depth review of EFAs. (P.S. I have no affiliation with or interest in the sponsoring company or with any other company or product mentioned in this book, in any manner whatsoever.)

[47] *Diabetologia* (1998 April; 41(4): 390–99).

[48] *Diabetologia* (1998, July; 41(7): 839–43).

noted the "marked synergistic interactions" between GLA and antoxidants.[49]

It is said that people are more likely to consume too much of omega-6 fatty acids and too little of omega-3s. A few scientists claim that typical American diets contain 20 times as much omega-6 as omega-3. Dr. Artemis Simopoulos says that human beings in the beginning evolved consuming a diet having approximately equal amounts of omega-3 and omega-6 fatty acids but that with the advent of vegetable oil consumption, the **balance** has **tipped** strongly to the latter.[50]

The relative **deficiency** of omega-3 acids in diets is particularly troublesome for PNers, and seems to be getting increasing recognition. A paper in the *Journal of Nutrition,* stated that "in humans with neuropathy or impairment of the immune system, significant deficits of omega-3 EFA have been found."[51]

Another study in the same journal, performed later in 1998 in Marseille, France, compared the feeding of olive oil and of **fish oil** (a source of omega-3, as noted) to small animal models in which diabetic neuropathy had been induced. The investigators said their data suggested that fish oil therapy "may be effective in the *prevention* of diabetic neuropathy [my emphasis]."[52]

---

[49] *Diabetes Research and Clinical Practice* (1999 Sep; 45 (2–3): 137–46).

[50] *American Journal of Clinical Nutrition* (1999 Sep; 70 (3 Suppl): 560-S-569-S).

[51] *Journal of Nutrition* (1998 Feb; 128 (2): 427S-33S).

[52] *Journal of Nutrition* (1999 Jan; 129 (1): 207–13).

There are different ideas on an appropriate ratio of gamma-6s, and the products that contain them, to gamma-3s and their associated host products. The Canadian Minister of National Health and Welfare in the early 90s was said to have recommended a ratio of six units of omega-6s to one unit of omega-3s. For someone on a 2000 calorie a day diet, the recommendation was 7 grams of omega-6s to 1.1 grams of omega-3s. The company that prepared the "bio FAQ" review previously referred to (Bioriginal Food & Science Corp.), gives the following suggestion: 2 grams of borage oil, 1–2 grams of flax oil and 2 grams of fish oil daily—roughly an even balance. They, and others, stress that the best solution might be to look for a blended oil product that combines EFAs.

In passing, I will mention a substance purveyed on the Internet which is claimed to do just that and to contain both omega-3 and omega-6 acids. One report (which can be seen at *http://emuszine.hypermart.net/pre_neuro.htm*) maintains that **emu oil,** in addition to providing general health benefits, is useful in treating peripheral neuropathy. This substance, available in refined form, comes from a flightless bird native to Australia. Emu oil is sometimes used topically; its proponents claim it is rapidly absorbed through the skin and relieves pain where applied. (Personally, I would be a little slow on this but it might be worth a try if all else fails.) By the way, emu oil is also sold for internal use as a dietary supplement.

Based on the above research, I have become an omega-3 believer and modified my own "EFA program" by adding

1000 mg (1 gram) of fish oil on a daily basis. (But boy, those capsules are big!)

2. Alpha-Lipoic Acid (ALA)

The beneficial effects of **alpha-lipoic acid** (**ALA**) supplementation for PNers were described in *Toes and Soles.* These include its action as a natural antioxidant, protecting nerves from oxidative damage and inflammation, as well as its ability to raise levels of the enzyme **glutathione,** itself a powerful antioxidant.[53]

ALA offers **dual antioxidant protection** in another sense because it is both fat and water soluble. Water solubility means that it works inside the nerve cell. Its fat solubility permits it to work outside the cell, at the membrane level. This double action on both sides of nerve cell walls is said to result in a stronger defense against damaging **free radicals.** (As mentioned before, these harmful molecular fragments are encountered by us every day through exposure to the sun's rays, automobile exhaust, smoke from various sources, and air pollution in general.)

The classic early study on the efficacy of alpha-

[53] Glutathione as an antioxidant itself protects nerves and virtually all other tissues in the body from oxidative damage by free radicals. A study in the *Journal of Trace Elements* (2000; 13: 105–11), maintains that although dietary supplements of this enzyme are available, they are not well absorbed by the GI tract and are therefore ineffective. In the Journal article Dr. J. Aaseth says that the antioxidant nutrients alpha-lipoic acid, vitamin C and vitamin E all help regenerate the body's glutathione.

lipoic acid for peripheral neuropathy, referred to as the **ALADIN study** (Alpha-Lipoic Acid in Diabetic Neuropathy), was performed in Dusseldorf, Germany, in 1995. The effects of ALA were studied in a 3-week multi-center, randomized, double-blind, placebo-controlled trial, in 328 non-insulin-dependent diabetic patients with symptomatic peripheral neuropathy. These patients were randomly assigned to treatment with intravenous infusion of alpha-lipoic acid at three dose levels (1200, 600, or 100 mg), or placebo. Neuropathic symptoms (pain, burning, *paresthesia,* and numbness) were scored at baseline and at each visit (days 2–5, 8–12, and 15–19) prior to infusion. Based on the study results the investigators said that using intravenous treatment at a dose level of 600 mg daily was effective in reducing symptoms of peripheral neuropathy without causing significant adverse reactions.[54]

Clinical evidence from various parts of the world continues to support the use of ALA for diabetic and other peripheral neuropathies. A randomized, double-blind study at the University of Zagreb in Croatia in 1999, concluded that after the daily administration of 600 mg of ALA to one group of diabetic patients and 1200 mg to another for a period of two years (65 patients in all), ALA "appeared to have a beneficial effect on several attributes of nerve conduction."[55] (The investigators did

---

[54] *Diabetologia (*1995 Dec; 38 (12): 1425–33).

[55] *Free Radical Research* (1999 Sep; 31(3):171–79). Results from clinical studies tend to be directed to and stated in terms of effects

qualify their opinion by saying that although neuropathic symptoms seemed to have improved over the 24 month study period, the "long-term response remains to be established.")

A three-week study performed in Dusseldorf, Germany, reached a similar conclusion. The patients with diabetic neuropathy enrolled there were given 600 mg of ALA three times daily. Researchers made the point that not only were neuropathy pain symptoms lessened but the nutrient was well tolerated.[56]

Russian investigator also found symptomatic improvement in a group of 29 patients with diabetic neuropathy after 14 days of ALA.[57]

Similarly, American investigators at the Mayo Clinic in Rochester, Minnesota, found peripheral nerve function improved in rats in which diabetic neuropathy had been induced, following the administration of ALA.[58]

---

of a particular therapy on subjective symptoms such as *paresthesia* and pain, or on objective parameters such as vibration threshold and nerve conduction velocity, and oftentimes on both subjective and objective "outcomes." Reference is made to fn 15 in Chapter 1 on the association of these measures.

[56] *Diabetic Medicine* (1999 Dec; 16 (12): 1040–43). To give perspective, I should report that another German study came to a different conclusion, finding "no effect on neuropathic symptoms distinguishable from placebo." They admitted, though, that their findings might have been off the mark because the various centers where the 509 patients in the study were examined were using different scoring methods [tsch!] (*Diabetes Care,* 1999 Aug; 22 (8): 1296–301). Interestingly, two of the investigators in this study were investigators in both the Zagreb and Dusseldorf studies just mentioned!

[57] *Zb Nevrol Psikhiatr Im S S Korsakova* (1999; 99(6): 18–22).

[58] *Diabetes* (1999 Oct; 48(10): 2045–51).

A more recent study delved into the nitty-gritty of the *way* ALA offers antioxidant protection.[59] Researchers in Germany investigated the effects of the nutrient on the body's **microcirculation system** for carrying oxygen to nerve cells. (This system consists of blood vessels such as capillaries with a diameter of less than 300 micrometers. Peripheral neuropathy is sometimes associated with a lack of blood circulation to the nerve cells.) The investigators concluded that microcirculation was benefited by the administration of either 600 mg or 1200 mg daily over a six week period. In technical terms they found that there was a decrease in the "time to peak capillary blood cell velocity,"—a marker in determining oxygen transport benefit.[60]

A study performed at the University of Texas Southwestern Medical Center at Dallas also examined the

---

[59] *Experimental and Clinical Endocrinology and Diabetes* (2000; 108 (3): 168–74).

[60] See also *Free Radical Research* (1999 Nov; 27 (9–10): 1114–22). Another recent study at the University of Michigan reported in *Diabetes* (2000 Jun; 49(6):1006–15), noted the "complex interrelationships among nerve perfusion, energy metabolism, osmolyte content, conduction velocity, and oxidative stress that may reflect the heterogeneous and compartmentalized composition of peripheral nerve." In particular the researchers said the studies implicated *oxidative stress* as an important factor in diabetic neuropathy.

One study, in concluding alpha-lipoic therapy "improves and may prevent diabetic neuropathy," indicated that "oxidative stress appears to be primarily due to the processes of nerve ischemia [reduced blood flow] and hyperglycemia auto-oxidation." (*In Vivo* 2000 Mar-Apr; 14(2): 327–30). An interesting paper concerning impaired blood flow with restricted oxygen delivery to peripheral nerves, implicates the accumulation of heavily glycated proteins within the arterial walls, resulting in "chronic vasoconstriction." *Free Radical Biology and Medicine* (2000 Feb 15; 28(4): 652–56).

manner in which ALA functions as an antioxidant, concluding it does so because "it decreases plasma—and LDL-oxidation."[61]

Finally a meta analysis in Germany (which pre-dated the Texas study) examined the results of 15 clinical trials.[62] The conclusion, based on all 15, was that short term (three weeks) treatment of diabetic neuropathy, using 600 mg per day of ALA, "appeared to reduce the chief symptoms" of neuropathy. Moreover, the preliminary data indicated to the investigators the "possible long-term improvement in motor and sensory nerve conduction in the lower limbs." The investigators emphasized that these 15 trials revealed a "highly favorable safety profile" for ALA.[63]

A recent paper, also from Germany and mentioned in the discussion of GLA, again acknowledged the benefits of ALA for the treatment of diabetic neuropathy: "Symptomatic therapy includes alpha-lipoic acid treatment, as the antioxidant seems to improve neuropathic symptoms."[64] (It should be noted that ALA is specifically approved for the treatment of diabetic neuropathy in Germany.)

---

[61] *Free Radical Biology and Medicine* (1999 Nov; 27(9–10): 1114–21).

[62] In a meta analysis or study, the results from a number of selected trials are combined in order to come to general conclusions. It is often used when a number of small trials give conflicting or statistically insignificant results.

[63] *Experimental and Clinical Endocrinology and Diabetes* (1999; 107(7): 421–30).

[64] *Fortschritte der Neurologie-Psychiatrie* (2000 Jun; 68 (6): 278–88).

Currently ASTA Medica is in Phase III trials with its ALA product, Thioctacid, for diabetic neuropathy.[65] Results should be available sometime in 2001.

Incidentally, in addition to painful sensory neuropathies, alpha-lipoic acid is useful with **autonomic neuropathies.** These disorders, which affect involuntary or semi-voluntary functions such as control of inner organs, are common among people with diabetes and have been reported to be present in up to 40% of Type 2 diabetic patients. Symptoms may include gastroparesis (a condition where the stomach is not emptying properly and characterized by nausea, vomiting, and abdominal distension), sexual dysfunction, low blood pressure when standing up (postural hypotension), and inability to sweat, as well as a variety of cardiac abnormalities. An earlier German study showed that alpha-lipoic acid caused a significant

---

[65] Most clinical trials are designated as Phase I, II, or III, based on the type of questions the study is seeking to answer for the FDA:

In Phase I clinical trials, researchers test a new drug or treatment in a small group of people (20–80) for the first time to evaluate its safety, determine a safe dosage range, and identify side effects.

In Phase II clinical trials, the study drug or treatment is given to a larger group (100–300) to see if it is effective and to further evaluate its safety.

In Phase III studies, the study drug or treatment is given to rather large groups (1,000–3,000) to confirm its effectiveness, monitor side effects, compare it to commonly used treatments, and collect information that will allow the drug or treatment to be used safely.

Most Phase III studies are randomized and blinded and typically last several years. Seventy to ninety percent of drugs that enter Phase III studies successfully complete this phase of testing. Once a Phase III study is successfully completed, a pharmaceutical company can request FDA approval for marketing the drug.

improvement in irregular heart rate in subjects with autonomic neuropathy.[66]

The **dosage range** for ALA is quite wide. Where used, practitioners recommend anywhere from 100–600 mg daily, with some going as high as 1200 mg.[67] You can look back at the dosages used in the clinical studies reported in this section to see the relative outcomes from different amounts. For myself, based on the reports I have seen, 600 mg daily is a good number whether taken at one time or, preferably, in divided doses. (I'll add that, in my opinion, ALA is a **must** for most PNers)

3. Acetyl-L-Carnitine (ALC)

The usefulness of **acetyl-l-carnitine,** an **amino acid** found in our body and frequently supplemented for therapeutic purposes, was discussed in *Toes and Soles.* As explained there, its claimed benefits, at least for those with diabetic neuropathy, are said to be based on the nutrient's **neuroprotective** and **neuroenhancing** properties. The rationale is that ALC raises **myoinositol** content in the nerves.[68] (Myoinositol is the active form of

---

[66] *Diabetes Care* (1997; 20: 369–73).

[67] In his March 2001 issue of *Health & Healing,* Dr. Julian Whitaker says that ALA is a "mainstay in a nutritional program for diabetics." He would go as high as 1800 mg daily for patients with diabetic neuropathies.

[68] Reduced levels of myoinositol have been observed in the sciatic nerves of rat models in which diabetic neuropathy has been induced. *Journal of Anatomy* (1999 Oct; 195 (Pt 3): 419–27). See also the *J Pharmacol Exp Ther* (1998 Dec; 287(3): 897–902): "ALC also

inositol, the latter a naturally occurring substance in the body necessary for the formation of **lecithin,** and which also aids in the breakdown of fats.) Additionally, ALC is considered a good **antioxidant.**

There seems to be a diversity of opinion now, though, as to how useful ALC is for someone with PN. Early studies were positive. For example investigators in Milan, Italy, working with diabetic animals, concluded in 1992 that ALC was potentially helpful in treating **autonomic neuropathies.**[69]

In 1995 other investigators at the University of Chieti in Italy, reported that 31 patients injected with one gram of ALC daily for 15 consecutive days, experienced reduced pain from diabetic neuropathy.[70]

The following year another group of researchers from Milan were less enthusiastic, concluding that ALC probably represented "only a co-factor" in the "clinical picture of human diabetic neuropathy."[71]

---

increased the myo-inositol as well as the free-carnitine content without affecting the sorbitol content. These observations suggest that there is a close relationship between increased polyol pathway activity and carnitine deficiency in the development of diabetic neuropathy and that an aldose reductase inhibitor, TAT, and a carnitine alog, ALC an, have therapeutic potential for the treatment of diabetic neuropathy."

[69] *International Journal of Clinical Pharmacology Research* (1992; 12(-6): 225–30).

[70] *International Journal of Clinical Pharmacology Research* (1995; 15 (1): 9–15).

[71] *Journal of the Peripheral Nervous System* (1996; 1(2): 157–63). This (mostly) same group seemed to reverse themselves the following year, at least with respect to one sub-population of people with PN.

Another contingent of Italian investigators went even further the next year in throwing a blanket of doubt over the benefits of ALC. Referring to the famous Diabetes Control and Complications Trial (DCCT) and the so-called Stockholm studies, they acknowledged that careful maintenance of near-normal blood glucose levels was the best approach to "primary and secondary prevention of peripheral neuropathy." ALC, aldose-reductase inhibitors (discussed in *Toes and Soles* and later in this book), gamma-linolenic acid, and antioxidants as a class, were all considered of "poor efficacy and often with significant adverse effects," in their view.[72]

The Japanese and the English appear to be in the opposite camp, investigators in those two countries both finding at least some merit in the use of ALC for treating peripheral neuropathy. The Japanese compared the effects of ALC and an aldose reductase inhibitor (known by its acronym, TAT) on neural functions in rats where diabetic neuropathy had been induced. They concluded that

---

They there concluded, after studying ten patients with HIV-induced peripheral neuropathy who were treated with .5 to 1 gram of ALC for three weeks, that "acetyl-L-carnitine can have a role in the treatment of pain in distal polyneuropathy related to HIV infection." The investigators cautioned, however, that "further double-blind, placebo-controlled studies" were required to confirm their results. *Journal of the Peripheral Nervous System* (1997; 2(3): 250–52).

[72] *Drugs* (1997 Sep; 54(3): 414–21). Clearly certain aldose-reductase inhibitors have caused problems for many people, with some ARIs even having been withdrawn from the market or from further testing, as will be later discussed. Throwing all antioxidants into the same heap seems extreme to me, however, based on so many other research results to the contrary.

both substances had "therapeutic potential for the treatment of diabetic neuropathy."[73]

In a paper presented in *Drug Safety,* two English clinicians reviewed the techniques for management of peripheral neuropathy in people with HIV infections. In their view, ALC and nerve growth factors such as recombinant human nerve growth factor (to be discussed later) are "agents that can helpfully assist" in managing PN.[74]

There you have it—somewhat of a mixed bag, with the preponderance of evidence, or at least claims from these studies, leaning in the direction of embracing ALC for PN treatments.

But what's a body to do, with all this confusion? Well the answer, for this one, is nothing, at least at this time. And I personally think that unless your PN stems from HIV or possibly diabetes, I would not consider adding ALC to a supplement program until there is more proof it would help. (But if one is of a mind to take a tad anyway the recommendation repeated in *Toes and Soles,* for therapeutic purposes, was 1500–3000 mg daily under the supervision of a physician.)

Two Natural Products

Following are a couple of natural substances not mentioned in *Toes and Soles,* said by some to provide relief for

---

[73] *Journal of Pharmacological Experimental Therapy* (1998 Dec; 287 (3): 897–902).

[74] *Drug Safety* (1998 Dec; 19(6): 481–94).

peripheral neuropathy. I was a little reluctant to include them because of the lack of documentation for PN use, but then I recalled that didn't really stop me from talking about such matters as chelation, hyperbaric oxygen therapy, or magnets, in *Toes and Soles.* Each of those modalities seemed to help some people in spite of anyone being able to explain in a totally satisfactory way just why that could be.

My philosophy, as set forth in my first book, is to bring to PNers' attention every strategy or approach that has at least good anecdotal support for effectiveness in dealing with our common malady. If the use of a particular therapy is backed by solid clinical studies or trials, great. But just because no one is willing to put up money for a particular study or trial—and companies rarely will if they cannot protect a proprietary position—there is no reason, in my mind, to dismiss out of hand an approach that seems to be helping people. At the very least I say, **let us make up our own** undoctoral (should I day undoctored?) **minds** after we've heard whatever evidence is available.

Having said that, just why **bromelain,** discussed below, may work for some people is a *particular* mystery. However, there might be some factor lurking in those pineapples that medical science does not understand—it's happened before, you know. Anyway, my take is that if it seems to work for anyone, hallelujah! (and a tip of the hat to those who insist on double-blind studies for everything).

The second, with the mellifluent name, **sangre de grado,** is from the bountiful Amazonian rain forest where so many drugs have been found (such as epibatidine, a secretion from the poison dart frog which holds much promise, as mentioned in *Toes and Soles* and discussed later here). There is more of a scientific basis for this substance.

1. Bromelain

This is an **enzyme** derived from **pineapple cores.** It is said to have powerful **anti-inflammatory properties** and reportedly has also been used in connection with heart disease and as an aid in digestion. It is considered generally safe when used moderately but there are reports it can lead to increased heart rate. (Also it is said to interact with blood-thinning drugs, so caution is advised.)

Sometimes the stem of the pineapple is juiced together with a few slices of the fruit, and four ounces or so of the resulting liquid is consumed daily. Bromelain is also available as a supplement in 500 and 1500 mg tablets.

There are people who swear bromelain has reduced or eliminated their neuropathic pain but I can find no studies which support that use. Be that as it may, it could be worth a try for some PNers, exercising proper precautions. I personally would make juice rather than buy more pills if I were to use bromelain in any form (which I do not plan to do, though I do like pineapples).

2. Sangre de Grado

Spanish explorers named the blood-red sap produced from a fast growing tree, **sangre de grado,** or blood of the dragon. It had been used for hundreds of years before the time of the conquistadors as an herbal remedy by Indians living in the Amazon River basin. It is still widely sold in Peru for diarrhea, gastrointestinal discomfort, and ulcers.

In fact, clinical studies show that the sap has a number of uses both topically and internally. It performs, for example, as an **analgesic,** quieting the firing of pain signals to the brain from sensory nerve fibers.

In a clinical trial in Louisiana (as reported in *Natural Science,* May 15, 2000), pest control workers were said to have found relief from a variety of insect bites and stings within 90 seconds. The investigators found that sangre de grado offered pain relief and alleviated itching and swelling symptoms for up to six hours.

A study performed at the University of Antwerp in Belgium found that the sap stimulated wound contraction and helped in forming new collagen and regenerating skin.[75]

Still another study performed at the Department of Pediatrics and Center for Cardiovascular Sciences at the Albany Medical College, New York, concluded that sangre de grado is a "potent, cost-effective treatment for gas-

[75] *Journal of Natural Products* (1993 Jun; *5* (*6*): 899–906).

trointestinal ulcers and distress via anti-microbial, anti-inflammatory, and sensory afferent-dependent actions."[76]

The possible benefits of sangre de grado to PNers, according to Dr. John Wallace of the University of Calgary, are based on the facts that "it not only prevents pain sensations, it also blocks the tissue response to a chemical released by nerves that promotes inflammation." Wallace claims there is no other substance which shares these two ends. He is so enthralled with the therapeutic prospects of this herb that he thinks "every medicine cabinet and first aid kit in North America will one day be stocked with medicines containing the sap."

There is still much research being performed on sangre de grado in the course of new drug development. For proprietary reasons much of this has not been disclosed to the public. It seems likely in the future, though, that we will hear a good deal more about the "blood of the dragon" as products are brought to market.

In concluding this chapter, I want to pass along the suggestions of Dr. Lark Lands from her forthcoming book, *Positively Well: Living with HIV as a Chronic, Manageable, Survivable Disease,* which she has kindly permitted me to set forth here. Although her book is directed principally to HIV-related neuropathy, her insights on nutrient therapy would seem generally applicable to other neuropathies as well:

---

[76] *American Journal of Physiology. Gastrointestinal and Liver Physiology* (2000 Jul; 279(1): G192–200).

For those wishing to try an integrated approach to reversing neuropathy or preventing its worsening with nutrients, those listed below are probably the most useful. Beginning with the fatty acids, alpha-lipoic acid and gamma linolenic acid, and the amino acid acetyl-L-carnitine, would probably be ideal since they are the nutrients whose effectiveness for diabetic neuropathy, and to a lesser extent HIV-associated neuropathy, is the most supported by research. For the most aggressive approach, which may well be the one most likely to succeed, all of these might be combined. With either approach, the following dosages might be reasonable to try: biotin (5–20 mg/day may be necessary), choline (400–800 mg of choline citrate or 1000–3000 mg of phosphatidylcholine, 3 times per day), inositol (500-2000 mg of myoinositol, three times per day), gamma linolenic acid (240 mg, 2–3 times per day), alpha-lipoic acid (200–400 mg, 3 times per day), B6 (50–100 mg/day in the form of pyridoxal-5-phosphate, or a combination of pyridoxine hydrochloride with pyridoxal-5-phosphate would probably be an appropriate starting dose, although higher dosages, of perhaps 100 mg, three times per day, might be required for treatment of some neuropathies), B12 (1000 mcg of B12, 3–7 times per week, preferably via nasal gel or subcutaneous or intramuscular injection, would probably be appropriate for most of those with neuropathy, with the frequency of dosing dependent on current symptoms), folic acid (1600 mcg, 3 times per day), niacin (25–50 mg, 3 times per day), thiamine (50 mg, 3 times per day), acetyl-L-carnitine (500-1000 mg, three times per day), and magnesium (500-1000 mg/day with one meal per day may be useful; best to take magnesium separately from calcium as they compete for absorption).

The Norwegian authors of a much cited study, "A Multidisciplinary Approach to Diabetic Neuropathy Treatment," Yngve Bersvendsen and Stan Angilley, focused on nutrient supplementation, have also been kind enough to share their latest thinking with me. Their suggestions are as follows:

1. As long before breakfast as possible, take one capsule of evening primrose oil containing 130 mg of GLA, and one tablet of alpha-lipoic acid—100 mg.
2. With breakfast, a "daily dose" of multivitamins/multiminerals, and two capsules of "Cardiovascular Research" magnesium taurate. (I asked them what this substance was all about and was told it yields a combination of magnesium and taurine, the latter being an amino acid which readily forms complexes with base metals—sort of a chelating process.)
3. An hour before lunch, one capsule (50 mg) of carnosine,[77] and one vitamin E capsule.
4. Two hours after the evening meal, on an empty stomach, one capsule of evening primrose oil (130 mg of GLA); 300 mg of alpha-lipoic acid in a time-release tablet; one tablet of "Alacer Supergram II" (mineral ascorbates including zinc and yielding 1 g of vita-

[77] Carnosine, also known as L-carnosine—but not to be confused with L-carnitine—is known mainly as an anti-aging supplement. It is a naturally-occurring combination of two amino acids found in concentrated amounts in long-lived cells such as in neuronal tissues. It is a water-soluble antioxidant thought to be a natural counterpart to lipid-soluble antioxidants such as vitamin E; as such it has been found to increase vitamin E levels in small animals. It also plays a part in neurotransmission and, as a heavy metal binder, chelates ionic metals. However, its most important contribution to diabetics is its anti-glycosylation effect.

min C); and 1 capsule of "Twinlab rice tocotrienol." (Tocotrienols are a particular form of vitamin E that act as "HMG-CoA reductase inhibitors, this substance being a key enzyme responsible for producing cholesterol in the body.)

I asked them whether they would make any changes in this regime in connection with non-diabetic neuropathies. They said that in their opinion the GLA plus alpha-lipoic acid combination was important because of the "trophic support" provided, but that the rest "may not be relevant."

I am totally convinced that following a good nutrient supplementation program is one of the best things—probably the very best thing—a PNer can do for symptomatic relief. My own was set out in *Toes and Soles.* At that time it consisted of daily amounts of:

- one vitamin B complex capsule ("B-50," containing 50 mg of B1, 50 mg of B2, 50 mg of Niacin, 50 mg of B-6, 400 mcg of folic acid, 50 mcg of B12, 50 mcg of biotin and 50 mg of pantothenic acid);
- 1000 mg of vitamin C;
- 400 IUs of vitamin E;
- 100 mcg of B12 (which was in addition to the above);
- 60 mg of alpha-lipoic acid;
- 1000 mg of evening primrose oil;
- 50 mg of zinc;
- 50 mcg of selenium; and
- one multivitamin/multimineral supplement taken mainly for the trace minerals (e.g., 20 mcg of sele-

nium, 2 mg of copper, 2 mg of manganese, 150 mcg of chromium; and 75 mcg of molybdeum).

Based on what I have learned since, particularly as a result of research for this book, I have made a few changes, namely:

- adding 1000 mcg of vitamin B12 sublingually in a methyl form;
- increasing the vitamin E to 800 IUs;
- adding 1000 mg of fish oil (for the gamma-3);
- adding 250 mg of magnesium;
- adding 30 mg of grape seed extract (for antioxidant protection);
- decreasing the evening primrose oil to 500 mg; and
- eliminating the 50 mcg of selenium (I figured I was getting enough in the multivitamin/multimineral supplement).

I still will be doing some tinkering—it probably would be a good idea to take more alpha-lipoic acid than factored in above, for instance, and to move to the benfotamine form of B1 sometime, but I'm already making Walgreen's the success story of the year. In the meanwhile, I can tell you, based on the above combination, SOMETHING IS WORKING![78] The problem is, I don't know exactly *what* it is. There surely must be some synergy involved among

[78] I can skip one of my 300 mg Neurontin capsules, scheduled 3xdaily, and often not even realize it. As recently as when I wrote *Toes and Soles,* there would be a pain penalty to pay for ever missing taking one.

all these supplements so I'll stay basically with what is outlined here, mindful of the growing body of evidence supporting the use of these nutrients.

Incidentally, try finding a doctor you can work with who is *sympatico* with your developing a nutrient program and who is knowledgeable enough to help you.[79]

---

[79] My wife told me, after reading this section, that she had just run into someone who had purchased *Toes and Soles* for her husband and asked whether the ideas in the book had helped her husband's peripheral neuropathy, particularly the ideas dealing with nutrient supplementation. The lady replied that her husband had mentioned nutrients to his doctor, and that product of many years of medical training said simply, "nutrients don't help, you just have to wait for the nerves to die." That kind of ignorance is inexcusable; it fortifies my desire to get the information in these two books into more hands as soon as possible.

Chapter 5

Updating Alternative/ Complementary Therapies

Many of us continue to seek treatments that don't involve gobbling up chemicals which might make us feel worse than before, or slathering ourselves with greasy concoctions which can sometimes burn (and who really knows what they might be doing to us under the skin), or having our blood exchanged for a new supply which we can only hope doesn't contain anything worse than we already have, or possibly being electrocuted or paralyzed by new or experimental nerve stimulation or nerve blocking techniques. (And to think that we often have to sit in a doctor's reception room for the better part of our remaining lives waiting to get an illegible prescription which we have to trust the pharmacist can decipher without substituting something that might kill or maim us for sure!)

I'm exaggerating, of course—but really, is it any big surprise that so many of us PNers are willing to try alternative treatments, considering how conventional therapies have failed?[1] Most of us have had chronic pain so long (that's what makes it chronic) that we're ready to give a go to anything that has any reasonable chance of succeeding.

A lot of others apparently feel the same way. According to a study reported in the American Chronic Pain Association, a survey of 1000 patients with chronic pain found 78% willing to try new treatments, with two thirds saying their nonprescription pain medicine was not "completely" or "not very" effective and 52% making the same observation about their prescription medication.[2] A re-

---

[1] Professor Clifford J. Woolf of the Harvard Medical School, writing on "Neuropathic Pain: Aetiology, Symptoms, Mechanisms, and Management," said in a rather devastating swipe at the allopathic approach to neuropathic pain:

> "[P]harmacotherapy for neuropathic pain has been disappointing. Patients with neuropathic pain do not respond to non-steroidal anti-inflammatory drugs and resistance or insensitivity to opiates is common. Patients are usually treated empirically with tricyclic or serotonin and norepinephrine uptake inhibitors, antidepressants, and anticonvulsants that all have limited efficacy and undesirable side-effects. Neurosurgical lesions have a neglible role and functional neurosurgery, including dorsal column or brain stimulation, is controversial, although transcutaneous nerve stimulation may provide some relief. Local anaesthetic blocks targeted at trigger points, peripheral nerves, plexi, dorsal roots, and the sympathetic nervous system have useful but short-lived effects; longer lasting blocks by phenol injection or cryotherapy risk irreversible functional impairment and have not been tested in placebo-controlled trials. . . . There is no treatment to prevent the development of neuropathic pain, nor to adequately, predictably, and specifically control established neuropathic pain." *Lancet* (1999; 353: 1959–64).
>
> His views, though perhaps unnecessarily grim, make the case even stronger for the implementation of the nutrient strategies discussed in the last chapter and in *Toes and Soles,* and the use, or at least the consideration, of therapies in this chapter.

[2] *The ACPA Chronicle* (2000 Nov; 18(3): 5).

cent survey by American Specialty Health and Stanford University School of Medicine reported that two out of three Americans now use acupuncture, herbal medicine, chiropractic, or other complementary and alternative therapies.[3]

This chapter has additional information on a few of those treatments that seem to work—at least for some of us. They often are employed as adjunctive or complementary therapies, meaning they are used in tandem with conventional treatments.

Acupuncture

This twenty seven hundred year old therapy, rooted in classical Chinese tradition, is based on the belief that **channels of energy** (**qi**) flow through the body. There are 12 of these channels or "**meridians,**" and each is named after the body part it is believed to influence. When this **energy flow** is impeded, disease results, according to Eastern belief. However, if hair-thin needles of varying lengths are inserted at specific points along the meridians and then perhaps twirled (with heat or an electric current sometimes applied to the needles), the energy flow will resume, returning health to the stickee.

The Western view, on the other hand, has simply been that nerves are **stimulated** by these needles, causing the **release** of **beneficial chemicals.** Researchers recently

---

[3] But not everyone thinks they should. The American Medical Association maintains that "there is little evidence to confirm the safety or efficacy of most alternative therapies."

demonstrated that acupuncture acts by first lowering blood pressure and normalizing heart function, which then causes the brain to release endorphins, the body's natural painkillers.[4]

Acupuncture continued to receive mixed reviews in studies published after *Toes and Soles* was written. You may recall that in one investigation reported earlier in this book, in the section on tricyclic antidepressants, acupuncture came off no better than amitriptyline or placebo in measures of pain relief. However, in a more recent PN study acupuncture did much better. Investigators used what was called "**electro-acupuncture,**" (referred to by some as ALTENS, or acupuncture-like transcutaneous electrical nerve stimulation, discussed in Chapter 3 under "Direct Nerve Stimulation"). Non-invasive skin electrodes were placed on leg acupuncture points of seven patients with HIV-related peripheral neuropathy, and low-voltage current was administered for 20 minutes every day for 30 days.[5] The investigators reported improvement in the condition of all seven. The patients also said they felt much better and reported feelings of increased physical strength.

---

[4] *American Journal of Physiology* (1999 Jun; 276(6 Pt 2): H2127–34).

[5] *Journal of Alternative and Complementary Medicine* (1999 Apr; 5(2): 135–42). Since meridian points were involved this *is* technically an acupuncture study although it deals with a subject akin to TENS therapy. Because of the confusion involved in nomenclature in these instances, one investigator suggests that a more appropriate term for acupuncture is "meridian therapy," encompassing all methods used to treat an acupoint. *AACN Clinical Issues* (2000 Feb; 11(1): 97–104).

In a case study of three patients with diabetic neuropathy who were given both **nefazodone** (a serotonin reuptake inhibitor) and acupuncture, the investigators found a marked and positive synergistic effect with two of the patients.[6] Nefazodone was given to all three first, resulting in a slight reduction in pain and other sensory symptoms as measured by a visual analog scale. However, when acupuncture therapy was added (six treatments, two at each visit), self-ratings for numbness, *paresthesia,* and pain fell dramatically for two of them, but only inconsequentially for the third. A follow-up indicated that for the two, the acupuncture benefits lasted "at least an additional six months."

The Mayo Clinic, in a July 20, 2000, review of acupuncture, pointed out that the National Institutes of Health has recognized acupuncture as an effective treatment for chronic pain, including the pain of neuropathy. (In a December 15, 2000, study entitled "Achieving Pain Relief Without Medication," the Mayo Clinic again acknowledged acupuncture as a valid therapy.)[7]

---

[6] *American Journal of Psychiatry* (2000 Aug; 157(8): 1342–43).

Some statisticians maintain that for case studies to have much validity, there should be at least five dealing with a particular subject, making for a "case series." Alas, we live in an imperfect world and will often have to do with less.

I like the comment that when a couple of doctors get together and happen to find a couple of similar outcomes, they are inclined to say later, "we see the same thing over and over again."

[7] In China, acupuncture is used not only for pain, but to treat various ailments and cure diseases. However, there is little evidence of its ability to do so. In the West acupuncture is used primarily to relieve pain or to help overcome nausea and vomiting and sometimes withdrawal from addictions or alcohol.

In a major review of the literature on acupuncture and chronic pain, results were examined from 51 previous studies. They were found positive for acupuncture in 21, negative in 3 and neutral in 27. Three-fourths of the studies received a low-quality score, and low-quality trials were significantly associated with positive results meaning that where the protocols were not tight or tightly administered, the outcomes were skewed in acupuncture's favor. Six or more acupuncture studies, however, were "significantly associated" with positive outcomes even after adjusting for study quality. The investigators concluded overall that "there is limited evidence that acupuncture is more effective than no treatment for chronic pain; and inconclusive evidence that acupuncture is more effective than placebo, sham acupuncture or standard care."

Thus even though the National Institutes of Health, as reported above, and the World Health Organization, as reported in *Toes and Soles,* have both gone on record saying that PN pain responds favorably to acupuncture treatment, there is a respectable body of evidence that it is only so-so at best. From my own vantage point, just based on anecdotal reports I've come across, more people seem to have been disappointed by acupuncture (as I was) than to have found benefit. Still, it apparently does work for some and might be worth a try.

Exercise

Next to making certain we are receiving the proper nutrients in an adequate amount, the most important thing a PNer can do is **exercise,** in my opinion.

Of course it's a natural reaction for many people to stop exercising when they get neuropathy; even the idea of getting re-started can be difficult for some. But we have to realize that once we stop exercising we are going to lose muscle strength and flexibility. And even though exercising won't reverse our neuropathy, it will keep our muscles in good working order, help improve our circulation and control our weight. Not only that, regular exercise will improve our digestion, permitting better absorption and use in our bodies of those all-important nutrient supplements.

Obviously any particular exercise program will depend on the age, general health and level of physical fitness of the PNer. Although exercise in the right amounts and of the right kind, helps just about anybody with peripheral neuropathy, it provides particular benefits for those with diabetic neuropathy. For those PNers it can result in improvements in glucose control, insulin sensitivity and blood pressure control.[8]

---

[8] The Joslin Diabetes Center, in a paper "Exercise for the Health of It," lays out the following benefits for those with diabetes:

> "Exercise can lower the blood sugar and improve the body's ability to use glucose. With regular exercise, the amount of insulin needed decreases.

Toes and Soles mentioned a number of exercises that can be undertaken by most PNers, including **walking,** the use of **stair-stepping, elliptical gliding** and **recumbent bicycling machines.** Since that book was published I have been reminded that there is another good activity for PNers: **rowing.** Certainly that is easy on the feet. Moreover you don't have to worry about balance because, just as with recumbent bicycles, you're sitting down. If you're not a member of a health club (and you do not fancy being out on the water), you can usually pick up a new rowing machine for several hundred dollars for home use, less of course for a used one.

Some of the very best work-outs for PNers still take place in the water. These exercises are particularly helpful because weight is taken off the feet and legs, and good resistance to muscle movement is provided.[9]

For those unable to do more, even sitting in a chair

Exercise can also help reverse the resistance to insulin that occurs as a result of being overweight. There is an increase in the number of insulin receptors improving the body's ability to utilize insulin.

Exercise improves risk factors for heart disease and decreases the risk of heart problems, which is a major health concern for people with diabetes. This includes the reduction of low density lipoprotein cholesterol (LDL), or bad cholesterol, which forms plaque that obstructs blood vessels.

Exercise promotes the good cholesterol, high density lipoprotein cholesterol (HDL), which is protective against heart disease. Blood pressure is also lowered through exercise and exercise has been shown to improve mild to moderate high blood pressure.

Exercise, when combined with a meal plan, has the ability to control Type 2 diabetes without the need for other medications.

Regular physical exercise and activity provides an effective way for a person with diabetes to manage their blood sugars."

[9] An excellent book, *The Complete Waterpower Workout Book: Program for Fitness, Injury Prevention, and Healing* (Random House

and performing light resistance exercises such as with a stretch band or with light weights, may help build and maintain muscle strength.

The special risks that those with Type 1 diabetes encounter exercising (as well as a few Type 2s) was noted in *Toes and Soles.*[10] One other particularly important caution should be observed in the case of those of either type having **diabetic autonomic neuropathies,** according to medical practitioners. This disorder can affect several systems necessary for the body's adjustment to exercise, particularly the **cardiovascular system.** Careful testing to evaluate **autonomic function** and to determine **exercise capacity** is extremely important with respect to these PNers; sudden death and myocardial ischemia have been attributed to "cardiac autonomic neuropathy."

Other precautions for those with diabetic neuropathy appear in a Position Statement from the American Diabetes Association on "Diabetes Mellitus and Exercise":

> There are several considerations that are particularly important and specific for the individual with diabetes. Aerobic exercise should be recommended, but taking precautionary measures for exercise involving the feet is essential for many patients with diabetes. The use of silica gel or air midsoles as well as polyester or blend

---

1993), may be ordered at the MedPress web site, *www.medpress.com.* Several other recommended exercise/physical therapy books are listed there as well.

[10] *The Physician and SportsMedicine* journal published a good paper dealing with all of this entitled "Exercise and Diabetes Control," in its April 2000 edition (Vol.28, No. 4).

(cotton-polyester) socks to prevent blisters and keep the feet dry is important for minimizing trauma to the feet. Proper footwear is essential and must be emphasized for individuals with peripheral neuropathy. Individuals must be taught to monitor closely for blisters and other potential damage to their feet, both before and after exercise. A diabetes identification bracelet or shoe tag should be clearly visible when exercising. Proper hydration is also essential, as dehydration can affect blood glucose levels and heart function adversely. Exercise in heat requires special attention to maintaining hydration. Adequate hydration prior to exercise is recommended (e.g., 17 ounces of fluid consumed 2 h before exercise). During exercise, fluid should be taken early and frequently in an amount sufficient to compensate for losses in sweat reflected in body weight loss, or the maximal amount of fluid tolerated. Precautions should be taken when exercising in extremely hot or cold environments. High-resistance exercise using weights may be acceptable for young individuals with diabetes, but not for older individuals or those with long-standing diabetes. Moderate weight training programs that utilize light weights and high repetitions can be used for maintaining or enhancing upper body strength in nearly all patients with diabetes.[11]

---

[11] The American College of Sports Medicine (ACSM) recommends that, for all individuals who have the capability of doing so (including those with diabetes who have passed medical examinations), aerobic physical activity should be performed a minimum of three to five days a week, for 20 to 60 minutes at 55 to 90% of maximal heart rate. For individuals not as well conditioned, they say that exercise can be done at the lower intensity level for a longer duration, at least until a higher level of fitness is achieved. Individuals with Type 2 diabetes should especially be encouraged to progress to a higher total duration of exercise (e.g., one hour daily) to facilitate fat loss, according to ACSM.

On the subject of feet and exercise for the PNer, the following ideas appeared in a paper concerning peripheral neuropathy in cancer patients. As modified here, I think there are some common sense thoughts for anyone with painful PN:

1. Standing in a confined space for a long period can contribute to neuropathic pain;
2. Sitting in a recliner makes pain worse;
3. Taking short walks and then elevating the feet help with pain;
4. Walking a little further each day and then giving your feet and legs a massage will cause pain to subside;
5. Exercise barefoot now and then, stretching the soles and spreading the toes;
6. Use a treadmill or stationary bike at the slowest speed and work very slowly up to faster speeds. Be cautious about treadmills and other mechanical exercise devices if you have decreased sensation in your feet or legs, or any balance problems;
7. The right dose of exercise should do no more than leave you pleasantly tired the next day.

Incidentally, the Neuropathy Association in New York publishes an excellent booklet on exercising. A copy may be obtained by contacting the Association at 1-800-247-6968. If you are not already a member, join up when you make your call! You will be rewarded in many ways—newsletters, the use of the bulletin board, the "Neuropathy Store," etc.

Hyperbaric Oxygen Therapy (HBO)

As I write this I am looking at a story which appeared in the *Washington Post* in April 1999, entitled, "Oxygen Therapy Joins Medical Mainstream." The writer said HBO (and she wasn't referring to the television entertainment channel) was formerly regarded as a "cure looking for a disease."

Her story concerned a diabetic who was at risk of having a foot amputated because of a wound which became infected so badly that gangrene had set in (a situation faced by more than a few PNers with diabetic neuropathy). After 50 or so sessions in a **hyperbaric oxygen** chamber his wound, which had been three and a half inches long and one inch wide in the beginning, was reduced to the size of a dime, according to the story.

The idea behind HBO is that pure oxygen introduced into a special chamber where the subject is seated, at a pressure several or more times ordinary atmospheric pressure, will permeate the body's tissues and restore circulation where blood flow had previously been restricted or reduced. Exposure to this massive infusion of oxygen permits every cell in your body to be flooded with a hundred times the oxygen it normally gets, according to HBO proponents. Several studies have shown the benefits of this therapy for peripheral neuropathy.

In a three month investigation of drug-induced neuropathies in 22 HIV-infected patients, 17 of the 20 who completed it were reported to have shown "significant improvement."[12] All of them had been taking antiretroviral medication for at least 12 months and had symptoms such as numbness or tingling, lethargy, and a decrease in deep-tendon reflexes.

Another study concerned "peripheral neural conduction, motor and sensory, in diabetic patients treated with hyperbaric oxygenation."[13] The Cuban investigators found a disappearance of *paresthesia* as well as of distal pains and leg and arm cramps.

One study seems to indicate HBO treatments might be used to **regenerate nerves.** The sciatic nerve was intentionally crushed in a number of rat models, some of which were then exposed to a series of 45-minute treatments every eight hours with oxygen at various pressures.[14] The investigators found that the "regeneration distances" were "significantly longer" in animals exposed to hyperbaric oxygen than those that were not (i.e., that the nerve axons grew further in the HBO group), and concluded their report with a statement that "HBO treatment stimulates axonal outgrowth following a nerve crush lesion."

Magnets

Magnetic therapy remains one of the most popular alternative treatments for many ailments, including pe-

---

[12] *Journal of the National Medical Association* (1998 Jun; 90(6): 355–8).

[13] *Revista de Neurologia* (1999 May 1–15; 28(9): 868–72).

[14] *Experimental Neurology* (1998 Feb; 149(2): 433–38). (I don't have much affection for rats but this better-them-than-us procedure bothered me.)

ripheral neuropathy. Yet it has as many scornful debunkers as enthusiastic believers.

Those who find efficacy say that it may be because magnetic fields **generate heat, expand the blood vessels** and **increase blood flow**, thereby bringing oxygen and nutrients to the affected area as well as reducing toxins. There also is a theory that the magnetic field in some way alters the manner in which pain signals are sent to the brain.

Toes and Soles mentioned a major double-blinded, placebo-controlled study at Baylor University in 1997, often cited by the proponents of magnetic therapy, where 76% of patients with diagnosed postpolio arthritic and muscle pains claimed a decrease in pain from the use of active magnets, versus 19% with placebo.[15] One of the study's detractors, caustically challenging both its methodology and the parameters used to measure pain reduction,[16] performed a blinded study himself on patients with diabetic neuropathy.

---

[15] *Archives of Physical Medicine and Rehabilitation* (1997 Nov; 78(11): 1200–3).

[16] Letter to the Editor, *Archives of Physical Medicine and Rehabilitation* (1998 Apr; 79(4): 469–70). To show he is even handed, Dr. Michael I.Weintraub castigated the investigators in another study (Collacott et al., reported in *Jama* (2000; 283: 1322–25)) who had found *no* significant differences in pain or other outcome measures between permanent magnets and matching placebo devices among subjects with back pain of a mean 19 years duration. Weintraub raised a number of problems with the study, saying it contained sex and selection bias, that the intervention was weak, and that the binders which held the magnets in place raised "issues of slippage." He also said that "all magnets are not the same," and that some "generate a deeper field gradient penetration." Letter to the Editor, (*Jama* 2000; 284: 565).

Dr. Michael I. Weintraub of New York Medical College in Briarcliff Manor, New York, randomized twenty four patients to either magnetic foot pads or placebo insoles for four months.[17] The patients wore the pads 24 hours a day. At the end of the study period nine of the 10 with the magnetized pads who completed the study reported "a significant reduction" in pain, according to Dr. Weintraub, versus only three of the nine wearing the placebo pads. Foot pain did return when the use of the magnetic insoles was discontinued, indicating to Dr. Weintraub that the treatment was "palliative but not curative." He also said that because of the small size of his investigation, results should be regarded as merely preliminary to additional clinical studies. (At the time this was written there was reportedly a nationwide study being planned at 100 centers in 50 states to validate those results.)

There is a technology revolving around a device called the Magna Bloc which some PNers claim has provided them with significant and long lasting relief. The unit, which was described in *Toes and Soles,* is an array of four magnets arranged in a square configuration with alternating polarity. It is claimed to alter the walls of nerve cells, thereby suppressing the transmission of painful impulses to the brain.

Until quite recently medical practitioners at Vanderbilt University, where the unit was originally developed, had been fitting Magna Blocs on interested patients, but

---

[17] *American Journal of Pain Management* (1999 Jan; 9: 8–17).

reportedly are no longer doing so. However, I understand Magna Blocs may be purchased from Nikken distributors. I have attempted to learn more from Vanderbilt concerning the status of the devices but they seem shy about providing information (as they were when I wrote *Toes and Soles* and attempted, unsuccessfully, to quiz them about Magna Blocs).

Massage and Other Touch Therapies

These therapies are used to **stimulate nerves** and **muscles** and/or call into play the "body's natural life forces." The basic **massages** covered in *Toes and Soles* result in **improved blood circulation** which is said to **increase oxygen capacity** (by up to 15%, according to the Johns Hopkins newsletter, *Health after 50,* August 2000), allow **muscular systems** to **relax,** and produce more **pain killing endorphins.** Other therapies such as **reiki, Qigong,** and **therapeutic touch,** are said to beneficially **manipulate** the body's **energy field** in various ways, much like acupuncture, according to Eastern practitioners.

Clinical evidence for resulting benefits from any of these therapies is still scant though many people attest to receiving help from them. In one study on the use of foot massage with hospitalized cancer patients, 87 subjects were given 10 minute massages over an extended period. The investigators found that there was a "significant, immediate effect on the perceptions of pain, nausea and relaxation."[18] (We could have told them that!)

(A surprisingly different result—at least to me—was reported from a randomized, sham-controlled, double masked study testing the short term efficacy of a 45 minute vibration treatment for foot pain in HIV patients with peripheral neuropathy.[19] The vibration therapy was delivered using a portable platform foot pain unit. The researchers found "no statistically significant differences" between the vibration group and the sham group in terms of pain relief! I have to think they were talking about long-term benefit.)

On the subject of feet (a subject many of us think about a lot), *Toes and Soles* discussed a particular massage technique called **reflexology.** This involves using thumbs and fingers to apply pressure to points or zones in the feet (and sometimes in the hands) corresponding to points in the body, thereby producing an array of claimed physiological benefits. In a study of 23 patients hospitalized with breast or lung cancer, reflexology was performed on their feet for 30 minutes by certified reflexologists.[20] Following this procedure, the patients were said to have experienced a significant decrease in anxiety. Moreover, one of three pain measures used was reported to have shown that patients with breast cancer experienced a significant decrease in pain. One can only speculate whether this would have any implications for those

---

[18] *Cancer Nursing* (2000 Jun; 23(3): 237–43).
[19] *Pain* (2000 Feb; 84(2–3): 291–96).
[20] *Oncology Nursing Forum* (2000 Jan-Feb; 271(1): 67–72).

of us with peripheral neuropathy. (As I indicated in *Toes and Soles,* the procedure did not help me but, then again, different things work for different people.)

Two fairly recent studies examined the efficacy of **therapeutic touch (TT)** for pain relief. You may recall from *Toes and Soles* (I hope you have read that book, which certainly makes the discussions in this one more meaningful) that "therapeutic touch" is a bit of a misnomer; there is really no touching involved. Rather the therapist's hands hover over the body to sense the "energy field pattern" and then redirect the energy into areas where needed.

In a study of 82 elderly people with arthritis, patients were assigned to either a TT group or into one using "progressive muscle relaxation" (i.e., hands on) treatments.[21] The researchers found that pain, tension, mood, and satisfaction improved in both groups but that "mobility and hand function" were significantly better for the TT group. (It was also found effective for pain relief in the treatment of osteoarthritis of the knee in another study.)[22]

In a study of patients in the advanced stage of Alzheimer's, patients in another TT group received five sessions of TT lasting 12.4 minutes while those in the control group received five sessions of "simple presence" lasting 10.3 minutes.[23] Results as reported indicated that the discomfort levels of those in the TT group had de-

---

[21] *Nursing Science Quarterly* (1998 Fall; 11(3): 123–32).
[22] *Journal of Family Practice* (1998 Oct; 47(4): 271–77).
[23] *Infirmiere du Quebec* (1999 Jul-Aug; 6(6): 38–47).

creased significantly compared with those in the control group.

(If you might recall from *Toes and Soles,* however, a study reported in *JAMA* dealt rather harshly with TT. I personally think there must be a strong placebo effect for those who think TT provides benefits but then, who really knows?)

Psychotherapies

The use of **psychotherapy** techniques for pain relief seems to be increasingly popular. One reason would seem to be the desire of patients to become more intimately involved in their own treatments.

1. Biofeedback

Toes and Soles discussed the use of **biofeedback,** a procedure in which people learn to control their health by **monitoring reports** from their own bodies. Typically a device is used which picks up signals from muscles where electrodes have been attached to the skin. The device then emits a visual or audible signal when the muscles tense. The patient can minimize the blinking or beeping signals emitted from the device by relaxing, resulting in the appropriate internal body adjustments. In time, this sort of "mind over matter" technique becomes ingrained, in theory permitting the subject to regulate processes such as heart rate, blood pressure, muscle tension and emotions.

There have not been many clinical studies on the

subject.[24] *Newsweek* ran a story on biofeedback in their June 19, 2000, issue, stating that even though it is new, biofeedback is emerging as a tool to treat many neuropathic disorders. The writer of the article, who also is the author of the book, *A Symphony in the Brain: The Evolution of the New Brain Wave Biofeedback* (Atlantic Monthly Press 2000), said that some experts believe this sort of regular brain wave training improves blood flow to particular brain regions, promoting stronger connections between cells. After 20 or 30 sessions, the sought changes seem to persist, according to the writer.

One unusual study used biofeedback in a "postural stability" training program for elderly patients with diabetic neuropathy.[25] Training sessions were scheduled three times a week for four weeks during which the subjects received visual feedback while they were standing on platforms which were made to rock. After 12 sessions those who had undergone the training showed fewer falls and longer delays in time between the rocking and their falls, compared with a control group. (I don't know who should be the most congratulated—the investigators who talked these worthy people into subjecting themselves to

---

[24] The author of a paper, "Psychological Aspects of Neuropathic Pain," wrote that it was surprising so few studies investigating the impact of psychological interventions for pain relief have been conducted, given the positive evidence. He did point out that there have been some *case series* reported, primarily in the area of biofeedback. *Clinical Journal of Pain* (2000 Jun; 16(2 Suppl): S101–105). However, the lack of studies should not be so surprising if you ask who is going to pay for them?

[25] *IEEE Transactions on Rehabilitation Engineering* (1997 Dec; 5(4): 399–402).

all those pratfalls, or the subjects themselves for surviving them.)

Several web sites offer information on biofeedback. One which lists associations and treatment centers is biofeedback.net. The author of the *Newsweek* article just mentioned says that his favorite site is *futurehealth.org/BFfaq.htm.* You can also join a discussion group at *egroups.com/group/biofeedback,* if you would like to get more information or just trade ideas with others.

2. *Hypnosis*

Since 1958 **hypnosis** has been recognized by the American Medical Association as a legitimate form of medical treatment. The increasing acceptance of the technique as a therapeutic adjunct by physicians and health care professionals has resulted in its broader use both in hospital and outpatient settings.

Toes and Soles outlined the premise behind hypnosis: when a subject enters into a hypnotic subconscious state, tuning out the surrounding environment, he or she is more susceptible to suggestions. ("I do not hurt, I do not hurt.")

One of the areas where hypnosis is sometimes used is in the management of cancer pain. In a review of various randomized, controlled studies of five different nonpharmacologic techniques (acupuncture, massage therapy, hypnosis, therapeutic touch, and biofeedback), the reviewers found that there was "much support for its [hypnosis'] use in the management of cancer pain."[26] The reviewers said the "evidence was either lacking or less clear for the other therapies examined."[27]

Researchers concluded in a meta analysis of 18 studies, that there was "a moderate to large hypnoanalgesic effect [i.e., of hypnosis], supporting the efficacy of hypnotic techniques for pain management."[28]

In a recent study comparing "standard care," "structured attention," and "self-hypnotic relaxation," for 241 patients undergoing invasive medical procedures, the clinicians said that "hypnosis had more pronounced effects on pain and anxiety reduction, and is superior, in that it also improves haemodynamic [relating to the mechanics of blood circulation] stability."[29] (It would be interesting to know just how that comes about.)

Dr. Jane E. Loitman of the Brown University School of Medicine, in an article entitled "Pain Management: Beyond Pharmacology to Acupuncture and Hypnosis," seems to hold the same view.[30] She said that "Patients [undergoing hypnosis] have reported feelings of heightened emotional well-being, deep relaxation, and reduc-

---

[26] *Cancer Prevention and Control* (1998 Feb; 2(1): 7–14).

[27] The authors of an article which appeared in *The Clinical Journal of Pain* on the "Psychological Aspects of Neuropathic Pain," said, in referring to an NIH study, that reviews of randomized clinical trials of hypnosis for chronic pain management, support its use only with chronic pain due to cancer. (2000 Jun; 16 Suppl (2): 101–105). The NIH study referred to had been performed in 1996.

[28] *International Journal of Clinical and Experimental Hypnosis* (2000 Apr; 48(2): 138–53).

[29] *The Lancet* (2000 Apr 29; 355 (9214): 1486–90).

[30] *JAMA* (2000 Jan; 283(1): 118–19).

tion of physical pain." She adds that "Research has not yet been able to delineate the mechanism underlying hypnosis' effect, but it appears to be more effective than placebo." (I can't imagine just what kind of placebo you would use to mimic hypnosis, but the premise makes sense to me. I think the real and unanswered question, though, may be what pain conditions, by types and degrees of severity, could effectively be dealt with using hypnosis.)

3. Meditation/Relaxation

Meditation and **relaxation** techniques are further examples of "mind over matter" ways of **controlling stress** and **anxiety,** and the disorders which result from those conditions. In fact, back in 1995 the National Institutes of Health found "strong evidence" that these techniques were effective in treating a variety of chronic states, from heart disease to migraines, lower back pain, and arthritis.[31]

An article at Healtheon/WebMD dated September 4, 2000, referred to two studies where it was found that chronic pain had been significantly reduced with the use of such techniques. Dr. Howard Fields of the University of California, San Francisco, explained in the article that meditation relieves the muscle tension which leads

---

[31] In "Dr. Dean Ornish's Program for Reversing Heart Disease," meditation is given the same importance for improving heart health as diet and exercise.

to pain. He also said meditation alters a person's response to pain.

Dr. Catherine Bushnell, Ph. D., at McGill University, was quoted in the same article as saying that relaxation techniques, including meditation and hypnosis, can allow people to tolerate pain they might ordinarily describe as unbearable. She added that relaxation techniques can change the way the brain responds to painful stimuli or how someone feels about it. According to Dr. Bushnell, meditation may also change the neural pathways that control physical pain sensations, dampening pain by "stimulating the inhibitory nerves that extend from the brain to the spinal cord, where they block the sensation of pain."

Stephan Bodian, author of the book *Meditation for Dummies* (Hungry Minds 1999), says it's the process of *practicing* meditation which makes it so helpful. He adds you don't need "any fancy equipment, tapes or the ability to sit cross-legged on the floor to meditate." He says that he just sits in a chair and tells himself to let go, visualizing somebody cutting a rope with knots in it. He points out there are many ways to meditate. You can count your breaths, focus on an image, or do whatever you're comfortable with—there is no right or wrong way. He suggests starting out with five minutes, gradually increasing the time.

Two recent papers published in medical journals indicate the benefits of meditation in particular ways. One discusses how the technique strengthens the body's immune system in combating infection and the growth of malignant tumors.[32] The other considers how, along with prayer, meditation reduces stress and improves mild hypertension.[33]

There are two therapies arising from the "arts" which perhaps ought to be mentioned here.

(a) Music Therapy

Music has had a place in medical practice throughout history and there now seems to be a growing interest in it as a therapeutic tool.

According to the American Music Therapy Association:

> The idea of music as a healing influence which could affect health is as least as old as the writings of Aristotle and Plato. The 20th century discipline began after World War I and World War II when community musicians of all types, both amateur and professional, went to Veterans hospitals around the country to play for the thousands of veterans suffering both physical and emotional trauma from the wars. The patients' notable physical and emotional responses to music led the doctors and nurses to request the hiring of musicians by the hospitals. It was soon evident that the hospital musicians needed some prior training before entering the facility and so the demand grew for a college curriculum. The first music therapy degree program in the world, was founded at Michigan State University in 1944. . . .
>
> Music is used in general hospitals to: alleviate pain

[32] *Seminars in Urologic Oncology* (1999 May; 17(2): 111–18).

[33] *Physical Medicine and Rehabilitation Clinics of North America* (1999 Aug; 10(3): 651–62).

> in conjunction with anesthesia or pain medication; elevate patients' mood and counteract depression; promote movement for physical rehabilitation; calm or sedate, often to induce sleep; counteract apprehension or fear; and lessen muscle tension for the purpose of relaxation, including the autonomic nervous system.

I found a couple of earlier studies referring to the therapeutic use of music. In one, the author determined that critical care patients experienced both **pain** and **anxiety relief** from music therapy.[34] The other analyzed the literature on musical therapy and found a number of reports supporting its use in the alleviation of pain in palliative (symptom management) care.[35] That study examined the presumed bases for reducing pain sensations, including a "psychological relationship" between music and pain (I must confess this was lost on me) and the fact that endorphins, the body's natural painkillers, are released when music is heard. (I think I understood that idea somewhat better.)

A recent study conducted in Norway pointed out that, historically, music has been linked to the treatment of mental illnesses, and has been used successfully to treat anxiety and depression and improve function in schizophrenia and autism.[36] According to the investigators, the combination of music with guided imagery and deep re-

[34] *Dimensions of Critical Care Nursing* (1995 Nov-Dec; 14(6): 295–304).

[35] *American Journal of Hospice and Palliative Care* (1996 Mar-Apr; 13(2): 43–49).

[36] *Tidsskr Nor Laegeforen* (2000 Apr 10; 120(10): 1186–90).

laxation has shown reduction of symptoms and increased well-being in chronic pain syndromes, whether from cancer or rheumatic origin. They also pointed to studies showing that music can improve function and alleviate symptoms in stroke rehabilitation, Parkinson's disease, Alzheimer's disease and other forms of dementia. They noted that music is well tolerated, inexpensive, and has few side effects.

An organization called the Institute for Music and Neurologic Function has recently been formed to conduct research, among other areas, in "music and recovery from nerve injury." The director of the Institute can be reached at 914-478-3700 (ext. 820), for further information concerning their programs.

Incidentally, I came across a new "therapy" which combines music with hypnosis, called "**high impact hypnosis.**" It is directed to people who say they are afraid of losing control in a hypnotic state. According to the English therapist who developed it, Lawrence Leyton, subjects remain fully conscious but totally relaxed during the self-administered therapy. Supposedly, specially orchestrated music uses repeat patterns and "digital delays which are incorporated with delays in the hypnotist's voice" which has been recorded, creating a "platform that maximizes the effect of the dialogue with the unconscious mind." A fuller explanation is offered in the February 2001 issue of *Positive Health* for anyone interested in trying something really different.

(b) Bibliotherapy

If the saying, "music tames the wild beasts," gives a sense of the theory behind music therapy, the inscription over the door of the Library at Thebes in ancient Greece, "Medicine for the Soul," may help convey the idea behind **bibliotherapy.** Each of these "therapies" is designed to promote a sense of **peace** and **tranquility,** thereby reducing tensions and fostering pain-free good health.

In a loose sense, bibliotherapy has been defined as the use of books to help stressed-out and depressed people solve problems. In a pilot program being funded by the British government, local health authorities, and a library's charity, doctors recently teamed up with librarians to deliver a "therapeutic course of novels to patients suffering from a range of ailments." Under the program, the librarian-bibliotherapist will scan a library's database to create a customized course of books designed to assuage each patient's particular malady. The program's organizer, herself a librarian, said the idea is for the bibliotherapist to talk to people, find out what kind of things they normally like to read, and then prescribe an individual list of books.

It appears any program such as that will not soon be adopted in the U.S. Officials at the American Library Association say they aren't accustomed to handing out "prescriptions for literary medicine."

Studies show mixed results for benefits of bibliotherapy. In one designed to determine who uses the procedure, and why, 68% of therapists queried in an Ontario community said they recommended books mainly to encourage self-help. The investigators concluded, after reviewing the information returned by the responders, that there was little evidence of therapeutic efficacy.[37] However, in a British study, "assisted bibliotherapy"—where selected patients were encouraged to manage their own symptoms as a result of book recommendations—*was* considered effective as a treatment for moderate anxiety problems.[38] (Maybe it just boils down to finding a good book to take your mind off your pain and/or other problems, which you probably can accomplish without assistance from anybody other than, perhaps, a helpful clerk in a book store.)

4. Prayer

The power of **prayer** as a medical therapy continues to be validated. Some of the benefits can certainly be explained by virtue of the **solace** and **reduction in stress** that ensues for the person who is praying. Other instances where health benefits may accrue to individuals as a result of intercessory prayer by others on their behalf, sometimes where the subjects are not even aware of the prayers, are not explainable, at least on any secular basis.

A six-year study was conducted at Duke University in which about 4000 senior citizens were asked whether they had any chronic health problems and whether they

---

[37] *Canadian Journal of Psychiatry* (2000 Sep; 45(7): 645–49).
[38] *British Journal of General Practice* (1999 Jan; 49(438): 47–48).

prayed, meditated or read the Bible.[39] The researchers found that those who said they never or rarely prayed ran about a 50% greater risk of dying during any given period than seniors who prayed or meditated at least once a month. The risk of death held even when factors such as smoking, drinking and social isolation were taken into account. This corroborates similar studies reported in *Toes and Soles.*

The subject of intercessory prayer—the praying for someone who may not be aware of the praying and where there is no or little logical possibility that the act of praying will itself provide therapeutic advantage—is gaining more attention. In one study, 920 patients admitted to coronary care were randomized to receive either remote intercessory prayer or nothing. The first names of patients in the prayer group were given to a team of outside intercessors who prayed for them daily for four weeks and never met the patients. The investigators concluded that "[intercessory] prayer may be an effective adjunct to standard medical care."[40]

In another study, the investigators reviewed randomized trials of intercessory prayer on behalf of people with various health problems.[41] One of the principal outcomes measured was death. The investigators found no evidence that prayer affected the numbers of people dying although they acknowledged their findings might have been flawed

---

[39] *Journal of Gerontology* (2000 Jul; 55(7): M400–405).

[40] *Archives of Internal Medicine* (1999 Oct 25; 159(19): 2273–78).

[41] *The Cochrane Database of Systematic Reviews* (2000; (2): CD000368).

by false assumptions. I thought the following statement from the study rather thought-provoking: "It could be the case that any effects [assuming a tendency toward positive outcomes] are due to elements beyond present scientific understanding that will, in time, be understood. If any benefit derives from God's response to prayer it may beyond any such trials to prove or disprove."

In an interesting study, investigators considered primary physicians' opinions regarding prayer and spirituality as they pertain to health.[42] Ninety-one percent of doctor respondents to a Mississippi survey considered prayer "an important treatment modality," but 50.6% rarely or ever discussed prayer with patients. Most who excluded prayer from their practices said they did so "to avoid imposing their beliefs upon patients."

---

[42] *Journal of the Mississippi State Medical Association* (2000 Dec; 41(12): 817–22).

Chapter 6

Experimental Therapies: Creeping Progress

The Holy Grail for PNers is the "true cure"—that is, the **complete restoration** of **neurological** and **physical functions** in our bodies and the consequent disappearance of all of our pain and other PN symptoms. If it is ever to be found it would appear most likely to involve either **nerve regeneration** or **cellular therapy,** or perhaps some combination of the two. These areas will be dealt with in this chapter.

Also included here are updates on other experimental work discussed in *Toes and Soles,* as well as reports on some new compounds which might provide better symptomatic relief for PN than treatments currently available.

As you will see, the path of progress in all of this is bumpy.

Neurotrophic Factors

Nerves in the peripheral nervous system have the inherent ability to **regenerate** themselves following lesions or other injuries, assuming the appropriate conditions are present. **Neurotrophic factors (NFs)** are large protein molecules produced by the body and responsible for the survival of neurons as well as for these "outgrowth" possibilities.

When, for example, **axons** (the long processes emanating from nerve cells which permit communication with other nerve cells) have been severely damaged by peripheral neuropathy, naturally occurring neurotrophic factors help the affected neurons grow their axons toward other neurons and restore functionality.[1] (These factors can also help repair myelin sheath which may have been damaged.)

This repair process is accomplished by the damaged neurons first selecting appropriate **target neurons.** These latter neurons secrete neurotrophic factor which directs "**growth cones**" at the tips of the advancing axons, to the connection.[2] To complete the process, structures must be made at the target for the release of neurotransmitters (chemicals) at the neuronal synapse (the

---

[1] This axonal growth proceeds at about one to two millimeters per day in man.

[2] "Eventual regrowth and reconnection with appropriate neuronal sites appear to involve both fiber-fiber and growth cone-target cell recognition." From "Nerve Regeneration," *Encyclopedia of Human Biology* (Academic Press 1997).

gaps between the neurons) so that the "electrical circuits" between the newly connected neurons are completed. This repair and restoration process is sometimes referred to as "**regeneration.**"

A number of neurotrophic factors have been discovered which **enhance** regeneration. Among the most promising are **nerve growth factor** (**NGF**) and **insulin-like growth factor** (**IGF-1**), both discussed in *Toes and Soles.* (These need to be synthesized in a manufacturing process since the brain, where endogenous [created within the body] production takes place, is often not capable of producing amounts sufficient for meaningful regeneration.)

1. Nerve Growth Factor (NGF)

The interesting potential of NGF to PNers is based on the fact that this neurotrophic factor supports the **small fiber sensory neurons** whose **degeneration** is associated with many pain symptoms of **sensory polyneuropathy.**[3] In this connection it has been found, for example, that levels of NGF are much reduced in patients with diabetes.[4] In one study it was demonstrated that reduced

---

[3] Another neurotrophic factor discussed in *Toes and Soles,* NT-3, has demonstrated efficacy for large fiber neuropathy, which can cause numbness and tingling.

[4] Italian clinicians have maintained that "deficiency of *several* neurotrophic factors, namely nerve growth factor (NGF) and IGF-I, has been related to the degeneration or impaired regeneration occurring in diabetic neuropathy [my emphasis]." *Hormone Research* (2000; 53(2): 53–67).

NGF in the skin of diabetic patients correlated with the presence of early signs of small fiber sensory neuropathy.[5] A scientist at Genentech, Inc., one of the leading proponents of NGF (at least until recently), has written that "in animal models of diabetes, depletion of endogenous NGF levels has been demonstrated in foot skin and skeletal muscle; these levels reduce further with increasing disease duration."[6]

Unfortunately, at least as measured by tools employed in the latest studies, the results to date for the use of recombinant (genetically recombined as opposed to endogenous)[7] nerve growth factor (rhNGF) in peripheral neuropathy, have been disappointing in spite of the theoretical promise.

First, in an earlier Phase II trial, which looked quite encouraging, investigators led by Dr. Stuart Apfel of the Department of Neurology, Albert Einstein College of Medicine, tested the effects of rhNGF in a study involving 250 people with diabetic neuropathy.[8] Of those, 82 received a placebo and 168 received rhNGF. All received injections three times a week for six months.

According to the investigators, patients taking the drug were found to be more responsive to heat, cold and

---

[5] "Diabetic Polyneuropathy," *Diabetes & Endocrinology Management,* 1999 Medscape, Inc.

[6] "Biological Actions of Nerve Growth Factor in the Peripheral Nervous System," *European Neurology* (1999; 41 Suppl 1:14–9).

[7] The submaxillary (salivary) gland of adult male mice is said to be the preferred source of *rhNGF.* Large concentrations are also found in bovine semen and guinea pig prostate tissue.

[8] *Neurology* (1998 Sep; 51(3): 695–702).

other sensations compared to those receiving a placebo. Of those receiving the drug, 75% responded positively when asked whether their symptoms had improved during the study, compared with 49% of those on placebo.

The most common side effect experienced was mild to moderate discomfort at the injection site. Because of this, most people receiving the drug correctly guessed they were receiving the drug and not the placebo. Most of the examiners also correctly guessed whether a particular patient was receiving the drug or placebo.

Because of the methodological flaw involving the unmasked placebo, another study was planned for diabetic neuropathy in which the placebo as well as the active injection would give patients mild discomfort at the injection site to keep everyone truly blinded.

In the meanwhile a Phase II double-blinded trial for nerve growth factor at 17 sites was conducted using 270 patients with **HIV-associated peripheral neuropathy.**[9] The patients were randomized into three groups, one receiving .3 micrograms of rhNGF per kilogram of body weight, one receiving .1 microgram per kilogram of weight, and the third, placebo. Fifty one per cent and 37%, respectively, of patients randomized in the higher and lower dose groups rated their neuropathic pain as "improved" or "much improved" at week 12 of the study period, compared to 23% among the placebo patients. At week 18, 36% of higher dose patients and 33% of lower dose patients rated their neuropathies as "improved" or

[9] *Neurology* (2000 Mar 14; 54(5): 1080–88).

"much improved" compared to 17% of placebo recipients. Moreover, sensitivity to pin pricks (a conventional test to assess neuropathy) was much improved in the two rhNGF groups as opposed to the placebo group.

Punch skin biopsies (a procedure to determine nerve densities) were performed in 60 patients, with no significant treatment effect being observed over the 18 weeks. No other changes in components of neurologic examinations, including vibratory sensibility, muscle strength, or deep tendon reflexes, were indicated, either.

The researchers said that this was the first trial involving the use of epidermal nerve fiber densities as a therapeutic outcome measure. They thought it "likely that regeneration or collateral sprouting of nerve fibers in the epidermis may take substantially longer than the 18 weeks of this study."

The most frequent adverse events were injection site pains, which were reported in 12 placebo recipients (15 total occurrences), 17 (25 occurrences) in lower dose rhNGF, and 36 (48 occurrences) in higher dose rhNGF subjects. The local injection site pain was dose-related, and usually lasted 10 to 20 days after each injection. The investigators concluded that about a third of the subjects were thus potentially unblinded by this adverse pain effect. Because of that, in similar fashion to the previous study concerning rhNGF with diabetic neuropathies, the researchers said that "in future studies, we may focus on physiologic outcomes or utilize an active placebo or some method of masking injection site pain to counter this."

After this study, Genentech, Inc., the corporate sponsor of both of these studies and the provider of the rhNGF used in the two of them, reportedly decided to withdraw from any further testing of the protein for **HIV-associated neuropathies** and concentrate instead on its possible use with **diabetic neuropathy.** (One report said the decision was based on the FDA's view that the results were not sufficiently positive to warrant further testing for the HIV syndrome.) Accordingly a Phase III randomized, double-blinded, placebo-controlled trial was pursued for **diabetic neuropathy.**[10]

In this study 1019 men and women with either Type 1 or Type 2 diabetes and a "sensory polyneuropathy attributable to diabetes," were evaluated over a twelve month period. Outcomes were measured by "impairment scores for lower limbs" (an overall score based on a graded battery of muscle strength, reflexes, and sensory testing), subjective patient assessments, and nerve conduction tests. To assure more effective blinding than occurred in the first two trials, a solution was chosen for the placebo which better mimicked the injection site hyperalgesia or pain associated with the rhNGF administration.

Based on the primary end points of efficacy (the impairment scores for lower limbs referred to above), 31% of the patients receiving the rhNGF were found to have improved, 38% worsened, and 31% remained unchanged. The rhNGF treatment group, in fact, did worse than the placebo group! Further, no beneficial effect of rhNGF versus placebo was observed for the majority of the secondary end points, according to the investigators. These in-

---

[10] *JAMA* (2000 Nov 1; 284(17): 2215–21).

cluded nerve conduction testing, subjective patient assessments, and the incidence of foot ulcers. The overall conclusion was that the trial failed to show a significant benefit for rhNGF when considering the outcome measures mentioned. However the investigators noted that there was a "modest but significant benefit" for severity of pain in the feet and legs.[11]

Clearly perplexed at the disappointing outcome, the investigators had several interesting observations:

> It is unknown whether NGF should be expected to improve neuronal function or just prevent progression of neuropathy in a clinical setting. *Each of the preclinical experimental models demonstrated that NGF has the ability to prevent neuropathy, not reverse it* [my emphasis]. Moreover, the doses of NGF used in those animal studies ranged from 1 to 10 mg/kg, administered between 3 and 7 times a week, in contrast to rhNGF administered at 0.1 µg/kg [sic], 3 times a week in our trial. Thus, the dose chosen for this study may be at the threshold or below the minimum dose needed to demonstrate efficacy. . . . It also is possible that our assessment was inadequate to detect a beneficial effect. All sensory measurements were performed at the toe. Considering

---

[11] Interestingly, several months before this study was reported in *JAMA*, Dr. Apfel, in an article, "Neurotrophic Factors and Pain," said that nerve growth factor "appears to be particularly important" with respect to pain. *Clinical Journal of Pain* (2000 Jun; 16(2 Suppl): S7–11). He went on to say significantly, that:

> "How NGF might improve neuropathic pain is not entirely clear. The time course for the improvement in symptoms is more rapid than might be expected if it were due to nerve regeneration or structural improvements in the degenerating neurons."

> the advanced neuropathy of our study population, improvement might have been detectable at more proximal locations where sprouting fibers are more likely to grow, and we might have missed it by restricting our examination to the big toe. In addition, the NIS-LL is not sensitive to small fiber sensory dysfunction, the neuronal population most likely to respond to rhNGF. This measure was chosen with the agreement of regulatory agencies since it was a validated instrument that can demonstrate a clinically meaningful change in functional status over time.

(I must say I found the observations that maybe something other than the big toe should have been examined, and that "impairment scores for lower limbs" were admittedly not sensitive to small fiber sensory dysfunction, which as stated by the investigators, is "the neuronal population most likely to respond to rhNGF," rather surprising.)[12]

Just before the publication of this book I spoke with Dr. Apfel, the lead investigator in this trial, about the future of NGF. He told me Genentech had decided to withdraw sponsorship of any further work with NGF because of the disappointing outcome of the Phase III trial. Dr. Apfel said he was hopeful, though, that another company might step in sometime in the future so that more

---

[12] See, for example, the paper "Human Studies of Recombinant Human Nerve Growth Factor and Diabetic Peripheral Neuropathy," where it was said study results "suggest that rhNGF specifically improves the function of small-fibre sensory peripheral neurons, which is consistent with its postulated mode of action." *European Neurology* (1999; 41 Suppl 1:20–26).

investigative work could be done. (I received the impression from him that he believed a longer trial period would have shown more positive results.)

I asked Dr. Apfel if symptomatic relief would be all that could ever be expected from NGF (which would be contrary to the hopes and expectations of many people looking for a total cure based upon the possibility of complete axonal and myelin sheath restoration). He said that not enough was accomplished in the trial to reach a definite conclusion on that question.

He also indicated that it would have been preferable if the study had been designed differently—to have focused, for example, more on the implications for small fiber neuropathy and to have chosen other measurement sites in addition to the big toe.

2. Neotrofin

NeoTherapeutics has developed an orally active small molecule (**AIT-82,** or **Neotrofin**) which reportedly passes across the **blood brain barrier** to produce **natural** neurotrophic factors where and when needed for nerve regeneration. (This barrier is a membrane which prevents **large molecules** such as typical NF proteins, when introduced into the blood stream orally or by injection, from reaching the brain or the cerebral spinal fluid.) AIT-82 is said to be able to selectively **turn on** genes and, when appropriate, activate **multiple genes** to **produce** different neurotrophic factors such as **NGF** and **NT-3** (discussed in *Toes and Soles*) naturally. The company claims this multiplicity of action is desirable because different factors have different mechanisms which together are able to produce greater neurological benefits than one alone.

NeoTherapeutics reported at the 30th Annual Meeting of the Society for Neuroscience in November 2000, that significant positive effects were seen in studies of peripheral nerve injuries in animals, without the detrimental effects of the increased pain frequently associated with *recombinant* nerve growth factor. On the 6th of November, 2000, the company announced it was discontinuing shorter-term clinical studies and would initiate a major one year study of AIT-82 for Alzheimer's disease while at the same time fund additional studies for other neurodegenerative conditions.

3. IGF-1

As explained in *Toes and Soles,* **IGF-1** is a neurotrophic factor produced in the **liver** and considered essential for normal growth of skin, bone, and nerves. It has been previously noticed that when **glucose levels** are high in people with diabetes, nerve cells produce less IGF-1 than normally. Deficiency of IGF as well as nerve growth factor has been related to the degeneration or impaired regeneration occurring in diabetic neuropathy.[13]

In a study reported in 1999, experimental diabetic *au-*

[13] *Hormone Research* (2000; 53(2): 53–67).

tonomic neuropathy was reversed in rats with the use of the factor.[14] The researchers had previously found that a distinctive type of structural change develops in diabetic rats—and man—which can be seen as large swellings forming into door-knob-like structures at the outermost tips of axons where nerve cells communicate with each other. In the study, diabetes was induced in rats over a six-month period—enough time to observe the occurrence of damage—and then daily injections of IGF-1 were given for two months. Compared with untreated animals, these rats had 80% fewer swollen nerve endings, and the swelling where it occurred tended to be less pronounced than in the untreated rats.

Robert E. Schmidt, M.D., the lead investigator of the study which took place at Washington University School of Medicine, said that he and his colleagues "made no attempt to control [the animals'] blood sugar and indeed, sought not to affect this value." (It is generally thought that control of blood sugar levels in people with diabetes is the most important factor in limiting complications of the disease.) He warned, however, that IGF-I does not represent "a replacement for the close control of blood sugar levels in the human diabetic."

IGF-I does present certain side effects when used at high dosages and could cause neoplasms (abnormal growths), according to Dr. Schmidt. Still he believes IGF-I may someday be an acceptable treatment for diabetic neuropathy, and perhaps for other nerve diseases.

---

[14] *American Journal of Pathology* (1999 Nov;155(5):1651–60).

As pointed out in *Toes and Soles,* researchers at Cephalon, Inc., have been studying IGF-1, mainly in amyotrophic lateral sclerosis (Lou Gehrig's disease). The company's most recent pronouncement of its involvement is as follows:

> Cephalon's drug development efforts in this area [of working with neurotrophic factors] focus on using the neurotrophic factor, IGF-1, to treat disorders such as ALS and peripheral neuropathies, where the projections of the damaged neurons lie or extend outside the blood-brain barrier and are therefore accessible to trophic factors, or in disorders such as multiple sclerosis, where the blood-brain barrier is compromised allowing trophic factors to cross into the CNS. In addition, Cephalon scientists are utilizing neurotrophic factors to further our understanding of the mechanisms of neuronal differentiation, death and survival to identify targets for innovative drug discovery.

Cephalon is supporting a recently undertaken "Trial of IGF-1 in the Treatment of Idiopathic Small Fiber Painful Neuropathy," at the Mayo Clinic.[15] (The investigators said that NGF was not employed because it had been shown to cause hyperalgesia—extreme sensitivity to pain.) Recombinant human IGF-1 (0.1 mg/kg/day) was being administered by subcutaneous injections in this double-blind study. A total of forty patients had been randomized for treatment or placebo for 6 months. The primary end-point was the subjective estimate of pain. Secondary end points included nerve conduction studies,

---

[15] Unreported in the literature as of this time.

computer assisted sensory examination, quantitative autonomic evaluation and quality of life scores. As of the time this was written four patients had significant improvement in symptoms, but their assignment to placebo or active drug was unknown. No patients had experienced significant worsening of symptoms; no serious adverse events had been encountered.

Another company working with IGF-1 is Aurogen. This company claims to hold patents covering the use of IGF and its **combination** with NGF to "treat diabetic neuropathy in mammals including humans." They say their scientists "developed the novel theory that the slow emergence of diabetic neuropathy over decades is due to: (i) a partial reduction in IGF activity as a result of diabetes, and (ii) a further gradual reduction in IGF activity with age over decades."

In comparing NGF with IGF, the company says:

> IGFs are likely to become the much preferred product to NGF. IGF but not NGF is expected to preserve sensory nerve regeneration as well as prevent motor neuropathy in diabetes. NGF can cause intense injection pain and may induce a chronic pain syndrome, but there is no evidence that IGF would. A cocktail of NGF and IGF may be best for some patients.

Dr. Douglas Ishii at Aurogen told me that a (yet unpublished) study at the University of Manchester found IGF treatments prevent abnormalities in a protein that determines the diameter of axons in diabetic rats. He said, though, that unfortunately his company has not been able to proceed with human clinical trials for IGF because "several million dollars are needed to produce IGFs to FDA specification."

Neuroimmunophilin Ligands

This forbidding name applies to a class of **small molecular compounds** which, proponents claim, holds particular promise for the treatment of neurological disorders. They have already been shown to enhance **neurite** (the in vitro equivalents of axons and dendrites) growth in culture.[16] In contrast to the neurotrophic factors just discussed, these substances readily cross the blood-brain barrier (similar to the reported action of AIT-82) and therefore may be administered orally.

Toes and Soles discussed **cyclosporin A** and **FK 506, neuroimmunophilin ligands** (**NL**s), which already have been used in humans as immunosupressant drugs. A recent paper points out that whereas both demonstrate **neuroprotective** actions, only FK 506 and its derivatives have clearly demonstrated an ability to exhibit significant **neuroregenerative** activity.[17]

The author, Dr. B.G. Gold at the Oregon Health Sciences University, said that a major breakthrough for the development of NLs for therapeutic purposes was the ability to **separate** the neuroregenerative property of FK 506 from its immunosupressant action. He said different receptor subtypes mediate the two activities and

---

[16] *Neuroscience* (2000; 100(3): 515–20).

[17] *Expert Opinion on Investigational Drugs* (2000 Oct; 9(10): 2331–42).

that the subtype which mediates nerve regeneration represents a "target for future drug development of novel classes of compounds for the treatment of a variety of human neurological disorders," including, he added, "peripheral nerve disorders."

Recently investigators conducted a review of six randomized controlled trials of FK 506 in nerve injury models of rats.[18] Measurements such as mean axonal area, axonal density and number of nerve fibers affected indicated a more than 50% increase in these measurements in all experimental animals where FK 506 had been administered, compared to controls.

Although these investigators concluded that the compound was a potent nerve growth stimulator, they said that further blinded studies in larger animal models, where axonal growth has to travel a greater distance from its injury site, would be desirable. They also wondered whether the risks of the toxic effects of FK 506 would generally be acceptable.[19] These investigators indicated that a convincing case for or against the use of FK 506 in nerve repair could not be made unless and until

---

[18] *Medjournal.com* (Archives 1999).

[19] These are said to include kidney damage, diabetes and high blood pressure. Also as many as 50% of patients will suffer infection, creatinine increase, headache, diarrhea or hypophosphatemia (a phosphate deficiency that results in bone defects). The nerve growth potential of FK 506 was confirmed in another study in which the authors proposed a further investigation using an experimental animal model incorporating a nerve conduit filled with slow release FK 506 at the site of the nerve gap or crush, thus decreasing the kinds of effects just noted. *The Canadian Journal of Plastic Surgery* (2000 May/Jun; 8(3): 97–100).

additional studies were performed to show risk/benefit ratios.

One of the NL compounds mentioned in *Toes and Soles* was GPI 1046, developed by Guilford Pharmaceuticals. As reported there, Guilford entered into a joint venture arrangement with a much larger biochemical company, Amgen, Inc., to further develop and market GPI 1046. Following experimentation with initial prototype compounds, Amgen and Guilford optimized a second-generation neuroimmunophilin ligand called NIL-A.

Amgen has completed Phase I clinical testing of NIL-A and in August 2000 began Phase II to evaluate the compound's safety and efficacy in the treatment of Parkinson's disease. (A representative of Amgen told me that as of the time this was written, reports were just beginning to come in on the Phase II study and that Amgen hoped to have publishable results later in 2001.) In addition, the partners are said to be working collaboratively to develop other neuroimmunophilin compounds for a variety of neurodegenerative diseases. According to Dr. Craig Smith, President & CEO of Guilford, these include potential treatments for disorders such as Alzheimer disease, multiple sclerosis, traumatic head and spinal cord injury, stroke, and *peripheral neuropathy.*

Another company working with neurophilin ligands is Vertex Pharmaceuticals. **Timcodar dimesylate** is their leading candidate in the neurophilin area. The company recently completed a study of the ligand in patients with diabetic neuropathy, assessing safety and pharmacokinetics over a 28-day dosing period. The product manager for Timcodar told me that Vertex is collaborating with Schering AG of Germany concerning further work with neurophilin ligands "for the treatment of neurological disease."

Incidentally, a company by the name of Jacobson Resonance Enterprises Inc., claims that a year-long study demonstrated that a low-level **magnetic field resonator** resulted in nerve growth and regeneration in mice.

Reportedly a team of researchers led by Dr. Brij Saxena, of Cornell University, used the "Jacobson Resonator" in applying low-level magnetic fields to mice sciatic nerves in vitro. The experiment was said to have verified that exposure to the unit's low-level magnetic fields triggered **growth** and **regeneration** of nerve sections in a culture medium. The researchers also reportedly found that nerves not exposed to the magnetic fields experienced nerve degeneration.

"At the end of the year we found, included in the new growth, myelin sheath, a structure responsible for normal nerve conduction of impulses," said Dr. Saxena. "These findings are especially important because the myelin sheath is the one part of the nerve that is commonly lost in neurological diseases. . . ."

A somewhat related development concerning nerve regrowth is based on the proposition that electrical fields enhance the healing of nerve, bone and other tissue. Although no one is exactly sure why, it is thought to have to do with the way calcium moves through cells in the presence of electricity. Now, according to a *Reuters* news story, it has been demonstrated that an **electricity-conducting plastic** has the ability to stimulate nerve regeneration when wrapped around severed nerves.

Called a "**polypyrrole,**" the special plastic is an **electroactive polymer.** Dr. Christine Schmidt at the University of Texas at Austin, has found the plastic to be safe when used surgically. She is developing a form of it which will dissolve naturally in the body after the nerve regeneration is complete.

Interestingly, the plastic seems to draw its electricity from ambient electric fields since Dr. Schmidt says that no outside current was used in experiments on rodents. In fact she plans on sending a mild electric charge to the plastic to see whether that will *further* speed nerve regrowth.

Although it may be difficult to see anything of practical significance to us from all of this, you never know where technology will lead. In the meantime if you see some PNer walking around with wires sticking straight out of his foot and a hopeful look on his face, that will prove there are those among us willing to try anything. (Note I said *his* foot and *his* face; women would never do anything that dumb. They would have known you need to attach metal hair curlers to the ends of the wires to pick up the whole electrical force field.)[20]

But now back to business.

---

[20] Just kidding, ladies. We know you are smarter than us. My wife proved it by pointing out that the electricity is *inside* our bodies. But in defense, she was in nursing where I guess they taught stuff like that; I was just a lawyer.

Cellular Therapies

This is a new approach to the treatment of neurological disorders, as well as of other disorders and diseases. Some think cellular therapies are such potentially powerful tools that they could redefine the practice of medicine in this century.

1. Gene Therapy

Proteins are directly involved in the chemical processes necessary to maintain life. Gene therapy involves supplying **DNA material** to cells for the manufacture of new **proteins** to replace proteins that may be missing or damaged.

This is accomplished by **packing genes** with the necessary material and **delivering** the genes to cells where the material is released and begins functioning—that is, making the particular protein required. Once this takes place the body can keep on making the needed protein as long as those cells live. In effect, the gene becomes the gift that keeps giving; obviously the therapy has advantages over simply administering a protein or a molecule.

Currently this treatment modality is being studied in a number of diseases, including cancer, peripheral vascular disease, arthritis, and neuro-degenerative disorders such as peripheral neuropathy. In the latter case it is at least theoretically possible to deliver **reparative genes** either directly to the peripheral nerves themselves or to the Schwann cells which produce the myelin coating protecting the nerves. Genes may also be delivered to other organs or tissues from which the beneficial effects of the transduced genes (i.e., genes in which the new DNA material has been incorporated) can be made available to the peripheral nerve system.

Certain key elements are required for successful gene therapy. First the relevant genes must be **identified** and **cloned.** Then, as mentioned, they must be carried or **delivered** to the targeted cell where they are to be **expressed** (i.e., where they manifest their effects by releasing the DNA).

In the delivery system, controlled **viruses,** referred to as "**vectors,**" encapsulate and carry the genes to the targeted cells. Viruses, from which deleterious matter has been removed, are usually used for this purpose because, over eons, they have developed extremely efficient means of targeting cells.

An excellent review of this technology appeared in a recent issue of *Drugs,*[21] by Dr. W. Walther and Dr. U. Stein at the Max-Delbruck-Center for Molecular Medicine, in Berlin, Germany, where they said:

> The efficient delivery of therapeutic genes and appropriate gene expression are the crucial issues for clinically relevant gene therapy. Viruses are naturally evolved vehicles which efficiently transfer their genes into host cells. This ability made them desirable for engineering virus vector systems for the delivery of therapeutic genes. The viral vectors recently in laboratory and clini-

[21] 2000 Aug; 60(2): 249–71.

> cal use are based on RNA and DNA viruses processing very different genomic structures and host ranges.

In discussing why particular viruses have been selected as gene delivery vehicles, the German clinicians said it was because of their capacities to carry foreign genes and their ability to efficiently deliver these genes:

> These are the major reasons why viral vectors derived from retroviruses, adenovirus, adeno-associated virus, herpesvirus and poxvirus are employed in more than 70% of clinical gene therapy trials worldwide. Among these vector systems, retrovirus vectors represent the most prominent delivery system, since these vectors have high gene transfer efficiency and mediate high expression of therapeutic genes. Members of the DNA virus family such as adenovirus-, adeno-associated virus or herpesvirus have also become attractive for efficient gene delivery as reflected by the fast growing number of clinical trials using these vectors. The first clinical trials were designed to test the feasibility and safety of viral vectors. Numerous viral vector systems have been developed for ex vivo and in vivo applications.

Concerning recent developments, they added that:

> Increasing efforts have been made to improve infectivity, viral targeting, cell type specific expression and the duration of expression. These features are essential for higher efficacy and safety of RNA—and DNA-virus vectors. From the beginning of development and utilization of viral vectors it was apparent that they harbor risks such as toxicities, immunoresponses towards viral antigens or potential viral recombination, which limit their clinical use. However, many achievements have been

made in vector safety, the retargeting of virus vectors and improving the expression properties by refining vector design and virus production.

In one recent study an **adenovirus vector**—which is similar to a cold virus—was used to deliver an encoded beta-endorphin (a naturally occurring pain reliever) gene to a rat's spinal cord via the fluid surrounding the cord.[22] (The spinal cord was said to have been chosen as the target for the gene not only because of ease of access but because pain can be effectively controlled at this location.) Within 24 hours the Schwann (sheath) cells surrounding the cord began secreting beta-endorphin, which eventually increased nearly 10-fold. The investigators ascertained a positive therapeutic effect by checking pain responses in the animal after the gene deliveries.[23]

In another example of successful gene transfer using adenovirus vectors, Korean clinicians were able to de-

---

[22] *Human Gene Therapy* (1999 May 1; 10(7): 1251–57).

[23] Adenovirus is said to be the only virus that works rapidly enough for many vector purposes. It is claimed that whereas most other vectors take 3 to 6 weeks to begin functioning, adenovirus vector starts to express genes within 24 hours. However, the future of the adenovirus as a vector, and gene therapy itself, was initially thrown in some doubt as a result of the death of a young, healthy volunteer, Jesse Gelsinger, in a gene therapy trial at the University of Pennsylvania in Philadelphia, in September 1999. He suffered a massive immune response to the carrier. Questions were subsequently raised as to whether the adenovirus vectors needed to be re-engineered to improve their safety. (See the article, "Gene Therapy on Trial," in *Science* (2000 May 12; 288: 951–57)).

In spite of the unfortunate Gelsinger experiment, gene therapy trials are continuing but with greater surveillance to make certain safety concerns are being met. (Incidentally, as of the time this was liver a "lacZ" gene (a gene which encodes a specific enzyme) into neuronal cells where **viral replication** had been purposely blocked.[24] The **expression** of the gene lasted long enough to accomplish nerve generation in a rat model.

Clinical delivery of a therapeutic gene for **peripheral neuropathy** was achieved in a 1999 study reported at the Annual Meeting of the Society for Neuroscience in Miami. Investigators demonstrated that a modified **herpes virus** can shuttle a therapeutic gene providing nerve growth factor not only to neurons that it typically enters, but also to non-neuronal cells. They also found that the newly manufactured NGF enters the bloodstream where it can travel to and potentially repair nerve-damaged sites throughout the body.

"These new findings are important for us to understand how this gene therapy may work in a clinical setting," remarked William Goins, Ph.D., assistant professor of molecular genetics and biochemistry at the University of Pittsburgh School of Medicine, where the study was performed. "Our results show that we could provide low-level, continuous production of nerve growth factor that could **circulate** throughout the body and po-

---

written, the Institute for Human Gene Therapy at the University of Pennsylvania, where the fatal trial was performed, has been banned from conducting clinical trials.) In fact the number of these trials is increasing, according to Inder Verma, editor-in-chief of *Molecular Therapy.* He sees no untoward long-term effects from the Gelsinger experiment on gene therapy but believes that scientists have become more "sensitized."

[24] *Molecules and Cells* (2000 Oct 31; 10(5); 540–45).

tentially **repair** nerves at sites far from where the gene is initially delivered. This therapeutic strategy could be extremely useful in the clinic."

In their studies, the Pittsburgh team used the herpes virus to deliver the gene to knee joints of rabbits and non-human primates. The researchers used two types of herpes virus, one engineered with a genetic component, or "**promoter,**" that turns on the NGF gene in neurons and one engineered with another promoter that turns on the NGF gene in cells other than neurons. Surprisingly, they found that both promoters were active, suggesting that the NGF protein was manufactured in non-neuronal cells, such as those found in ligaments and tendons within joints, as well as in neuronal cells.

Researchers at the Institute of Child Health, University College in London, recently pointed out that the herpes virus has unique advantages as a vector in terms of its large genome size and its ability to enter a latent state in neuronal cells.[25] They also said that considerable progress has been made in the effective **disablement** of the virus (to do away with its inherently harmful properties) while retaining its ability to deliver genes and to produce "long term expression of the foreign gene." They maintained that "although much remains to be achieved in the further disablement of the virus and its testing in rodent and primate models of human diseases," it is probable that herpes viruses will find particular use in otherwise intractable neurological diseases.

---

[25] *Histol Histopathol* (2000 Oct; 15(4):1253–59).

One of the limitations involved in vector-based gene therapy is the relatively short period that the delivered gene is permitted to do its work, or is expressed. For example, investigators in the study reported above concerning the "**transduction**" (the transfer of the genetic material) of the encoded beta-endorphin gene, said that production peaked after three to seven days and tailed off dramatically by day 15. A Swiss study describes a microneurosurgical technique where replication-defective viral vectors were injected into dorsal root ganglia rather than directly into the sciatic nerve.[26] Researchers said this permitted sustained expression for more than 100 days. More progress can be expected along this line.[27]

At the same meeting of the Society for Neuroscience held in New Orleans in November 2000, at which NeoTherapeutics reported on their AIT-82 product (just discussed), another important cellular development was presented. Findings were detailed in which spinal cord injuries had been treated using genetically modified cells that **secreted** the pain-relieving chemical, **serontin.** In that case genetically engineered cells were **directly implanted** into the area of injury in laboratory rats.

Senior author of the paper on this development, Claire E. Hulsebosch, Professor of Neuroscience at the University of Texas Medical Branch at Galveston, said

---

[26] *Proc Natl Acad Sci U S A* (2000 Jan 4; 97(1): 442–47).

[27] A recent investigation reported the use of **moth cell virus** in a gene transfer method called "baculovirus transduction," which supposedly will result in a more prolonged and efficient transduction. *Diabetes* (2000; 49(12)).

that "serotonin inhibits neurons that are in the pain pathway. In addition, serotonin helps locomotion." He added that the animals returned to their pre-surgical condition.

Gene therapy would appear to hold great promise for the treatment of peripheral neuropathy, particularly where used with neurotrophic factors to promote nerve regeneration.[28]

2. Stem Cell Technology

The ability of the body to **generate entirely new cells** to help treat diseases and disorders is based on the fact that so-called "**stem cells**" produce all the different types of cells that make up the body. If these master cells are isolated and cultured under proper lab conditions at an early stage, medical researchers say they may be able to use them to **replace** damaged or missing organs and tissue.[29]

Stem cells are extracted from **human embryos** or **aborted fetuses.** Approximately four days after fertilization a structure called the **blastocyst,** a hollow sphere of cells which become stem cells, is formed out of the embryo. Stem cells which have been removed from the blas-

---

[28] See, e.g., the *Journal of Neurotrauma* (1998 Jun; 15(6): 387–97): "The expression of growth-promoting proteins through adenoviral vector-mediated gene transfer may be a realistic option to promote peripheral nerve regeneration."

[29] Neither stem cell technology nor gene therapy should be confused with another relatively new technology called "xenotransplantation." This involves implantations of living cells from other species when human donors are not available, for example when an organ is needed or when animal cells may provide a unique benefit.

tocyst can be cultured and formed into other cells such as liver cells, red blood cells and nerve cells. In fact stem cells have the ability to **differeniate** into any of the more than 200 cell types in the human body.

Work based on their remarkable differentiation capabilities resulted in the technology being dubbed the 1999 "Breakthrough of the Year" by the prestigious magazine, *Science.* ("We salute this work, which raises hopes of dazzling medical applications and also forces scientists to reconsider fundamental ideas about how cells grow up." *Science,* December 17, 1999).[30]

It has been pointed out that a number of disorders, including those of a neurodegenerative nature, are associated with the death of specific cell populations which are not able to regenerate themselves. Important therapeutic values of stem cells come not only from their ability to overcome this failure by metamorphosing into the kind of cells required, but also their ability to self-renew and divide for sufficient periods to form the tissue required.

One example of their potential use might be the transplantation of healthy **heart muscle** cells to patients with chronic heart disease whose hearts no longer pump adequately. Preliminary work in mice and other animals has demonstrated that healthy heart muscle cells trans-

---

[30] Interestingly, the completion of gene sequencing of complex organisms ranging from the fruit fly to the human was cited by the same magazine as the "Breakthrough of the Year" the following year. (*Science,* December 22, 2000). The publication went on to say, in a burst of awe, that this one "might well be the breakthrough of the decade, perhaps even the century, for all its potential to alter our view of the world we live in."

planted into the heart successfully repopulate the heart tissue and work together with the host cells.

At the time this was written, Dr. Ole Isacson of Harvard Medical School and Dr. Ronald McKay of the National Institutes of Health, just reported they had "cured" Parkinson's in mice and rats, using stem cells removed from embryos of laboratory animals.[31]

In a report presented to the national meeting of the American Association for the Advancement of Science in February 2001, Isacson said mouse and rat embryonic cells, after careful processing, could be grafted into the animals' brains where they differentiate into replacements for cells killed by Parkinson's. Using a slightly different technique, McKay said his NIH lab had also prompted mouse embryonic stem cells to convert into cells free of the Parkinson's defect.

It is thought that **spinal cord injuries** might also be treated with stem cells. Injected soon after damage to the cord, the cells could mature and reconnect the severed nerves. Scientists speculate that the treatment might prevent or reverse paralysis in people who would ordinarily be confined to a wheelchair. Other potential neurological disease targets could include multiple sclerosis and peripheral neuropathy because cells could be grown

---

[31] More than a million Americans have been diagnosed with Parkinson's, a disease caused by the death of brain cells which produce dopamine, a key nerve chemical. When patients lose about 80 percent of these cells, they reportedly develop the classic Parkinson's symptoms: tremors and rigidity. Parkinson's can be treated with L-dopa, a drug that makes dopamine in the brain. But L-dopa is said to be effective for only a short time and after that the disease progresses.

to reline the protective coating of nerves and/or enhance axonal development.

At present, stem cells deemed capable of producing all of the various tissues in the body are derived from human embryos or aborted fetuses, as indicated. The use of stem cells from these sources, though, has given rise to major ethical concerns based on the sanctity of life.

In late August 2000, the National Institutes of Health (NIH), after taking into account thousands of comments (most of them negative), ruled that NIH funds may be used for research on stem cells only if they were derived from embryos *left over from fertility treatments.* The rationale is that this tissue is marked for destruction, anyway. The opponents of using stem cells derived in this manner are not satisfied with NIH's ruling, however, and have threatened legal action as of the time this was written.[32]

An approach possibly avoiding these difficult questions is the use of **adult stem cells.** These are cells already existing in our bodies that reproduce as needed to renew tissues. The problem here has been, though, to cause these cells to differentiate and grow into all the kinds of tissues as those "stemming" from embryos are able to do. It had been commonly thought, for example that "once a blood cell, always a blood cell."

In a feat many thought impossible, however, **bone**

---

[32] Nevertheless, according to a Reuters Health report dated 1/22/01, nearly two-thirds of Americans support federal funding for stem cell research.

marrow adult cells have been transformed into **neuron-like** cells in living animals.[33] This research is considered particularly significant because scientists had believed brain cells were the only ones capable of developing into nerve cells.

Researchers say that bone marrow cells, which are an easily available source of stem cells, could be used as an ample source of neurons that might need to be replaced as a result of neurological disorders. (There still remain questions whether these newly generated neurons would function as normal neurons and whether they can make appropriate connections with other cells.)

In another study reported at the Annual Meeting of the Society for Experimental Biology in San Diego in April 2000, scientists were able to produce mature **liver cells** from purified **blood stem cells** in mice.

Since there is so much controversy over using stem cells from embryos or fetuses, one might well ask why all efforts shouldn't be concentrated on adult stem cells. Following is what the NIH has to say in part:[34]

> Any attempt to use stem cells from a patient's own body for treatment would require that stem cells would first have to be isolated from the patient and then grown in culture in sufficient numbers to obtain adequate quantities for treatment. For some acute disorders, there may not be enough time to grow enough cells to use for treatment. In other disorders, caused by a genetic defect, the genetic error would likely be present in the patient's

---

[33] *Science* (December 1, 2000).

[34] "Stem Cells: A Primer," National Institutes of Health, May 2000.

> stem cells. Cells from such a patient may not be appropriate for transplantation. There is evidence that stem cells from adults may not have the same capacity to proliferate as younger cells do. In addition, adult stem cells may contain more DNA abnormalities, caused by exposure to daily living, including sunlight, toxins, and by expected errors made in DNA replication during the course of a lifetime. These potential weaknesses could limit the usefulness of adult stem cells.[35]

Putting aside NIH's concerns, it may be some while before marrow or blood-derived adult stem cell therapies can be fully tested in humans. Still scientists think results from animal tests are encouraging. The November 2000 issue of the *Mayo Clinic Health Letter* maintains that "if progress with blood and bone marrow transplants is any indication, stem cell research will someday help many people." Let's hope that PNers are included.

3. "Biologic Minipumps"

This technology involves the **implantation** of **neuronal cells** that have been specially modified for a particular purpose. They are **grafted** near spinal cord pain centers and secrete or "**pump**" selected **molecules** such as neurotransmitters, neurotrophins and peptides, on a continuous basis.

In one study, neuronal cells were grafted near the spinal cord in a rat model in which chronic neuropathic pain

[35] At the time this was written, President George W. Bush had just gone on record saying he prefers adult stem cell research, signaling he may move to block the other types.

had been induced.[36] The cells were **genetically modified** (in vitro) to secrete brain derived neurotophic factor before the transfer. The researchers found that the cells thus grafted were able to deliver NF for a sufficiently long period to "reverse the development of chronic neuropathic pain." They said that "such 'biologic minipumps' can be developed for safe use in humans."[37]

The technology, though still new and relatively untried, would seem to offer great promise. Researchers at the University of Miami School of Medicine, recently said, in decorous understatement, that "The development and use of cellular minipumps, immortalized cell lines bioengineered to secrete various antinociceptive [pain relieving] molecules for the reversal of neuropathic pain, makes cellular therapy a strategy for clinical use in the next few years."[38]

4. Nerve Cell Disablement

Scientists funded by the National Institute of Neurological Disorders and Stroke (NINDS) think it may soon be possible to reduce chronic neuropathic and inflammatory pain by **disabling** certain nerve cells that send pain signals to the brain.

As reported in *Science,* combining **substance P** with

---

[36] *Pain* (2000 May; 86(1–2); 195–210).

[37] See also *Cell Transplantation* (1999 Jan-Feb; 8(1): 87–101), reporting on the successful use of cell "minipumps" to provide inhibitory neurotransmitter GABA molecules to rats in which chronic neuropathic pain had been induced.

[38] *Journal of the Peripheral Nervous System* (2000 Jun; 5(2): 59–74).

saporin in a rat model inhibited the pain associated with nerve injury and significantly reduced sensitivity to stimuli associated with inflammatory pain.[39]

Researchers at the University of Minnesota injected a combination of substance P (a neurotransmitter known to stimulate pain receptors) and saporin (a neurotoxin) into the dorsal horn of the spinal cord in rats. Receptors for substance P—large molecules found on the surface of spinal cord nerve cells—served as portals for the compound's entry. Within days, the targeted neurons, located in the outer layer of the spinal cord along its entire length, absorbed the compound and were neutralized.

Researchers said the substance P/saporin treatment appeared to lessen the pain response both to thermal and mechanically induced pain and that the results seemed to be long-lasting.

They concluded that the small group of neurons that express substance P plays a critical role in communicating chronic pain information from the spinal cord to the thalamus, the brain's pain center, and that using specific receptors to introduce therapeutic compounds might pave the way for a new pain therapy.

Such compounds might be first introduced through a lumbar puncture, a technique commonly used for collecting spinal fluid, according to the researchers. The compounds would then serve to relay information through the spinal cord to the thalamus, thus blocking pain signals.

---

[39] *Science,* November 19, 1999.

"These findings are extremely important to the study of peripheral and neuropathic pain and our treatment of persons with persistent pain," says Patrick Mantyh, Ph.D., of the University of Minnesota and the Veterans Affairs Medical Center in Minneapolis, who led the study. "We were able to administer a potential treatment and specifically channel it to certain cells, disabling them. We can now focus on the biology of these cells and look at new ways of silencing these cells in other types of persistent pain."

"This discovery is critically important to our understanding of the pain process," says Cheryl Kitt, Ph.D., program director for pain at the NINDS. "Understanding pain pathway changes at the cellular level offers great potential for more effective treatment for pain."

Though the technique appears to work well in rats, cautioned Michael L. Nichols, a neurology researcher at the University of Minnesota in Minneapolis, there needs to be more research before it can be tested on humans, including tests on higher animals such as monkeys. However, he noted that humans, like rats, have the same substance P neurotransmitter that relays pain signals in the nervous system.

Some Promising (and not so Promising) Experimental Drugs

1. ABT-594

A tropical frog, "epipedobates tricolor," is the source of the toxic chemical **epibatidine.** This tiny creature has no natural enemies since a single frog is said to contain enough chemistry within its skin to kill a water buffalo!

As reported in *Toes and Soles,* chemists at Abbot Laboratories have converted this chemical into a powerful pain-relieving substance named **ABT-594.** The drug, said to be a "**neuronal nicotinic receptor agonist,**" is reported to be **200 times** more potent than morphine.

A 1999 study reported that ABT-594 had a demonstrated analgesic effect and an improved safety profile compared with epibatidine itself.[40] However, the drug raised some concerns as to **adverse side effects** in a study performed in England the next year where it reportedly was found to have produced hypothermia, seizures, and dose-dependent increases in blood pressure.[41] (The researchers found, though, that these effects could be attenuated with the co-administration of another drug called **mecamylamine.**) Shortly after that, ABT-594 was again compared with epibatidine in another English study, where both were found to reverse inflammatory and neuropathic hyperalgesia (increased sensitivity to pain), with ABT-594 displaying a "clearer separation between its motor and anti-hyperalgesia effects."[42]

A company representative at Abbot Laboratories told me that, as of the time this was written, Abbot was about to begin Phase II trials of their product for diabetic neuropathy. Progress thus continues, albeit slowly.

---

[40] *Biochemical Pharmacology* (1999 Sep 15; 58(6): 917–23).
[41] *Pain* (2000 Apr; 85(3): 443–50).
[42] *Pain* (2000 May; 86(1–2): 113–18).

2. *Agmatine*

This is a newly-identified **neurotransmitter** found in the brain and spinal cord. It has been shown to be effective both in reducing chronic pain symptoms and as a **neuroprotecter,** according to Donald Reis, M. D., Department of Neurology and Neuroscience at Cornell University.

In addition to being a neurotransmitter (a naturally occurring chemical which conveys pain signals) and neuromodulator, **agmatine** is also an "**endogenous ligand**" (no, not some kind of exotic lizard but rather a substance synthesized in the brain which has a strong affinity for one or more of the neuron receptors located there).

In a study at the University of Minnesota, synthesized agmatine was administered to rodents with spinal cord injuries and was found to have decreased hyperalgesia accompanying inflammation, as well as allodynia (touch evoked pain).[43] The researchers said that the evidence from both this and earlier studies suggested "a unique neuroprotective role" for agmatine in "processes underlying persistent pain and neuronal injury."

That conclusion was affirmed in another study reported shortly thereafter involving spinal cord ischemia (tissue anemia due to an obstruction of arterial blood flow) in a rat. The lead investigator concluded that "agmatine is an efficacious neuroprotective agent and that

---

[43] *Proceedings of the National Academy of Sciences USA* (2000 Sep 12; 97(19): 10584–89).

this naturally occurring non-toxic compound should be tried for therapeutic use after neurotrauma and in neurodegenerative diseases."[44]

The role for this substance has not been defined yet for peripheral neuropathy but these research results offer hope that some day it will find its way into the arsenal of compounds that could help PNers.

3. *Aminoguanidine (pimagedine)*

As noted in *Toes and Soles,* this compound is an **AGE,** or "**advanced glycation product.**" Clinicians have thought **aminoguanidine** prevents the accumulation of these glucose-modified proteins frequently associated with diabetic neuropathy.

In a study performed at the Department of Pathology at Japan's Hirosaki University School of Medicine (when it comes to research in diabetic neuropathy, the Japanese are covering all the bases), researchers explored how aminoguanidine **inhibits** neuropathic changes in diabetes compared with insulin.[45] They found that although there was some improvement in rat models, the substance was not nearly as effective in improving nerve conduction velocity as insulin.

Aminoguanidine was used in a study with baboons in a somewhat later study in Australia, and again was found wanting.[46] The treatments to the primates were

---

[44] *Neuroscience Letters* (2000 Dec 22; 296(2–3): 97–1000).
[45] *Diabetologia* (1999 Jun; 42(6): 743–47)
[46] *Diabetologia* (2000 Jan; 43(10; 110–16)

administered over a three-year period and reportedly had no effect on glycemic control or axon density. Also the treatments did not restore nerve conduction velocity or autonomic dysfunction in the diabetic animals. (In other words, it appeared the whole thing was just monkey business.)

I spoke with a representative of Alteon, Inc., a company which has been working with aminoguanidine (they refer to the compound as **pimagedine**) in other areas of diabetic complications. She told me Alteon has put any future plans for pimagedine on "the back burner" until additional financing is obtained. Instead she said the company is concentrating its energies and limited resources on another diabetic product it calls **ALT-711.**

Incidentally, ALT-711 is what is referred to as a crosslink breaker (AGEs ultimately form crosslinks with adjacent proteins, leading to a loss of flexibility and function in body tissues, organs and cells), and is in Phase IIA clinical testing to evaluate its effect on cardiovascular activity. Additional indications being evaluated are said to include non-obstructive uropathy (a disease of the urinary organs) and scleroderma (a usually slowly progressive disease marked by the deposition of fibrous connective tissue in the skin and often in internal organs).

According to the company's representative, ALT-711 could ultimately prove superior to pimagedine in treating neuropathies.

The disappointments with aminoguanidine/pimagedine illustrate quite clearly the risks inherent in experimental drug work. As *Toes and Soles* had related, studies performed in Scotland, Japan, and the United States all had shown that aminoguanidine might have potential in the treatment of *human* diabetic neuropathy.[47] Now it appears it can't even do the job with rodents or apes.

4. Memantine

Prospects continue to brighten for this investigational drug ultimately being approved by the FDA for peripheral neuropathy.

As discussed in *Toes and Soles,* **Memantine** is an orally administered compound which acts to **modulate** the N-methyl-D-aspartate ("NMDA") receptor by reducing the potentially damaging influx of excessive calcium ions.

Animal models have helped researchers discover that these receptors share a special relationship with neuropathic pain. It appears that continuous activation of NMDA receptors reorganizes pain-sensing circuits and leads to the super-sensitive quality of neuropathic pain. Agents that block or modulate the receptors also block or modulate pain in animals and humans. This action can restore functional neuronal impairment associated with a number of disorders, including chronic conditions of neuropathic pain, dementia, and Alzheimer's disease,

---

[47] As recently as mid-1999, it was reported that "therapies for distal polyneuropathies include metabolic treatments (e.g., aldose reductase inhibitors, **aminoguanidine,** gamma-linolenic acid, autoimmune therapies, and nerve growth factor)." *American Journal of Medicine* (1999 Aug 30; 107(2B): 17S-26S).

as well as acute conditions of traumatic brain injury and stroke.

The broad Phase IIB trial of Memantine *Toes and Soles* had mentioned, which was initiated in late 1998, was concluded with quite positive results. The developer and manufacturer of the product, Neurobiological Technologies, Inc. (NTI), reported outcomes at the Annual Meeting of the American Academy of Neurology in May 2000, in San Diego. Four hundred and seven people had participated in the double-blind, placebo-controlled study. Two dosage levels were compared against placebo, one of 20 mg daily and the other 40 mg daily, over an eight-week period. There was no significant difference between the 20 mg dose group and placebo. However, there reportedly was a 50% pain reduction experienced by 44% of patients in the 40 mg group.

Richard G. Pellegrino, M.D., chief investigator, said the study "provides a new alternative for treating diabetic neuropathy, a treatment with good efficacy and few side effects." He added that he expected the next step would be to design a Phase III study for diabetic neuropathy comparing the 40 mg dosage with placebo in 400 to 500 patients.

In the meanwhile, enrollment was completed in 2000 for a double-blind, placebo-controlled Phase II clinical trial of Memantine for AIDS-related dementia, funded by the National Institute of Health (NIH) and conducted by the AIDS Clinical Trials Group (ACTG). The primary benefit sought is "improvement of neurological function and peripheral neuropathy," according to the company.

In June 2000, Forest Laboratories, Inc., was granted rights for the development and marketing of Memantine in the United States for the treatment of neuropathic pain, Alzheimer's disease, and AIDS-related dementia.

As of the time this was written, Memantine appears to be a prime candidate for possibly broad use with peripheral neuropathy.

5. Pregabalin

In studies of rat models, **pregabalin,** a synthetic **GABA analog** (GABA—gamma-aminobutyric acid—is an inhibitory neurotransmitter which helps prevent nerves from "firing too fast"), has been found to reduce neuropathic pain.[48] Recent studies have considered whether it would have the same effect on humans and have sought to determine the relationship between **neural function** and **pain relief** associated with pregabalin.

In safety and efficacy studies, 584 patients with diabetic neuropathy of one to five years' duration were randomized to receive pregabalin or placebo three times daily.[49] Compared with placebo, pregabalin at both 300 mg daily and 600 mg daily reduced weekly mean pain scores "significantly." The drug likewise proved more effective than placebo on other measures, including sleep

---

[48] See, e.g., *Pain* (1999 Mar; 80(1–2): 391–98).

[49] Program and Abstracts of the 19th Annual Scientific Meeting of the American Pain Society; November 2–5, 2000; Atlanta, Georgia. Abstract 679.

interference scores. Adverse events in these studies were said to have been principally mild to moderate dizziness and somnolence; 31 patients withdrew because of side effects.

In an analysis of those studies, investigators found no direct relationship between pain and neural function.[50]

However, in at least a temporary setback for pregabalin, the drug's manufacturer, Pfizer Corp., halted clinical trials in early 2001 after a study indicated that it increased the incidence of **tumors** in **mice.** The company said it still expected the drug to win FDA approval (it has hailed the drug as a "painkilling leap, with the power of morphine") despite the setback, arguing there is no evidence that it causes tumors in humans.

(Both Pfizer and the FDA noted the anomaly that rats were not affected in the studies reported above. Pfizer spokeswoman Mariann Caprino said the company was going to do "another mouse study.")

6. Tiagabine (Gabatril)

Tiagabine joins a long list of other anticonvulsants—gabapentin, lamotrigine, topiramate, zonisamide, etc.—which were developed to treat epilepsy but which are being used or experimented with in peripheral neuropathy as well.

---

[50] Ibid., 678. In reaching this (to me) surprising conclusion, the investigators used a scoring system designed to provide a quantitative estimate of the severity of neuropathy in each patient at baseline (at the beginning) and at the termination of the study.

This compound is also said to work by **enhancing** the inhibitory neurotransmitter, **GABA.** It accomplishes this by blocking its reuptake into presynaptic neurons, increasing extracellular concentration of GABA and prolonging its inhibitory action. The result is that neural impulses which contribute to seizures are quieted.

Its possible use in dealing with neuropathic pain was considered in two studies dealing with animal models.[51] Results from those indicated that further studies in humans are warranted.[52]

Zigs and Zags

Two experimental drugs at the end of the alphabet — **zenarestat** and **zopolrestat**—known as **aldose reductase inhibitors,** have had their futures pretty well zapped by their manufacturer. They were both discussed in *Toes and Soles* as possibly offering some hope. A third experimental drug, **ziconotide,** may turn out to be a real

[51] *Epilepsia* (1999; 40 Suppl 9: S2–6); *Drugs* (2000 Nov; 60(5): 1029–52).

[52] Misha-Miroslav Backonja, M.D., mentions another possible anticonvulsant candidate—vigabatrin—for the treatment of neuropathic pain in his article, "Anticonvulsants for Neuropathic Pain Syndromes," *Clinical Journal of Pain* (2000 Jun; 16(2 Suppl): S67–71). I could find only one slightly relevant study concerning vigabatrin for this purpose. It was conducted in Brazil in 1999, and involved experiments with rat models in which a "constrictive sciatic neuropathy" was induced. The researchers noted a "possible analgesic effect" that was dose-dependent. *Arquivos de Neuro-Psiquiatria* (1999 Dec; 57(4): 916020).

zinger. A fourth alphabetical tail-ender, **zonisamide,** has recently appeared on the investigational scene and, according to preliminary reports, zounds zuper.

1. Zenarestat

As indicated in *Toes and Soles,* an accumulation of **sorbitol** is often found in diabetic nerve tissue which appears to upset the chemical balance in nerve cells and increase the severity of diabetic neuropathy. The enzyme or protein which produces sorbitol is called **aldose reductase.** To diminish excess sorbitol production, a class of compounds called aldose reductase **inhibitors,** or **ARI**s, have been developed over the last twenty years or so.

Toes and Soles detailed the difficulties ARIs have had in proving themselves as offering significant benefits for neurological disorders in spite of their theoretical promise. (There are currently no aldose reductase inhibitors available on the US market. Reports of liver toxicity resulted in the removal of **tolrestat** from all markets in 1996.)

Based on earlier clinical trials, one of the better candidates had appeared to be **zenarestat,** but its prospects were extinguished rather abruptly. In October 2000, Pfizer, the drug's U.S. sponsor, disclosed that it had halted further development because zenarestat was found to have potential **renal** (kidney) **toxicity** in some of the estimated 3700 patients participating in a Phase III clinical trial worldwide. The outcome was discouraging because nerve conduction tests in earlier studies had proven quite positive.[53] In spite of the adverse side effects which led to the discontinuance of development, nerve conduction results in the Phase III trial were favorable.

Interestingly, Japanese investigators, who just coincidentally happened to be employees of the company (Fujisawa Pharmaceutical) which first had developed zenarestat, later affirmed findings that the compound offered therapeutic potential. However, they side-stepped the renal toxicity issue.

2. Zopolrestat

The same company, Pfizer, which had abandoned zenarestat and was forced to discontinue—at least temporarily—trials of pregabalin, was disappointed in its study of yet another ARI, **zopolrestat.** (It had named this product **Alond.**)[54]

The 18-month multi-center trial with 431 patients with either Type 1 or Type 2 diabetes having diabetic

---

[53] Just prior to Pfizer's announcement, another study, this one a 52 week, randomized, double-blinded, clinical trial, found that sorbitol suppression accomplished by zenarestat resulted, dose dependently, in improved nerve conduction velocity and in significant increases in the density of small-diameter myelinated nerve fibers. *Neurology* (1999 Aug; 53: 580). As a kind of advance warning, though, the investigators noted that more than 80% suppression of nerve sorbitol content was required to stop or reverse the progression of diabetic neuropathy and that "potent [i.e., toxic?] ARIs" might be required.

[54] Lest one feel sorry for Pfizer because of its recent disappointments with neuropathic pain products, it should be noted that this research powerhouse was marketing *eight* billion-dollar products

neuropathies, had just gotten underway when *Toes and Soles* was written. Later reported data from the study indicated that changes in nerve fiber density based on biopsies—a key end-point chosen by the company to assess the outcome—were rather small in both the Alond and the placebo groups.

The company made the interesting, and telling, observation that "the data suggest that it may be very difficult, in clinical trials of *practical duration,* to demonstrate the effects of new drugs on the rate of nerve degeneration using *existing* measurement technologies [my emphases]."

Among the other ARIs discussed in *Toes and Soles,* little has occurred in the way of new developments. The Japanese still appear, though, to be interested in pursuing studies of the effects of these substances on diabetic neuropathy.

Epalrestat, dealt with in *Toes and Soles,* was evaluated at the Tottori University College of Medical Care Technology in Yonago, Japan, in a 36 month test with 22 subjects concerning its effects on "diabetic cardiovascular neuropathy."[55] The mean age of the subjects was 64.8 years and the mean duration of their diabetes, 7.8 years. The investigators concluded that long-term administration of this ARI was beneficial in even relatively older subjects with diabetes of long duration.

---

at the last count: Lipitor, Norvasc, Celebrex, Zoloft, Viagra, Diflucan, Neurontin and Zithromax. It also has a number of other drug candidates in the wings.

[55] *Diabetes Research and Clinical Practice* (1999 Mar; 43(3): 193–98).

The same ARI was found in another Japanese investigation to have "effectively reversed diabetic neuropathy."[56]

The indefatigable Japanese, apparently the principal champions of ARIs these days, have developed yet another candidate: **fidarestat.** True to their tradition, all the reported research comes directly out of the labs of the corporate developer. In the first investigation, fidarestat was compared with epalrestat and zenarestat as to effects on nerve conduction velocity.[57] With results that should be surprising to no one, investigators found "significant effects" on nerve conduction velocity that were "more potent than those shown by the other inhibitors." In a burst of enthusiasm they added that "Fidarestat suppressed sorbitol accumulation remarkably and continuously until 24 h after administration," while the "inhibitory effect by zenarestat declined in a time-dependent manner," with epalrestat having no effect whatsoever.

Perhaps because of their trail blazing work in the first study, the same corporate investigators were soon called upon again to assess (applaud?) the effects of **long-term** treatment with fidarestat. They found that following the administration of their company's product, demyelination and axonal degeneration were reduced to normal levels in rats whose diabetic neuropathies had been induced.[58] In conclusion they added that "long-term treat-

---

[56] *Clinical Nuclear Medicine* (1999 Jun; 24(6): 418–20).

[57] *Journal of Diabetes Complications* (1999 May-Jun; 13(3): 141–50).

[58] *Diabetes Research and Clinical Practice* (2000 Oct; 50(2): 77–85).

ment with fidarestat substantially inhibited the functional and structural progression of diabetic neuropathy," thereby doubtlessly earning themselves at least a holiday to Mt. Fuji.

(Just prior to publication of this book, another Japanese ARI study was reported, this one involving a substance known as **tetrazolacetic acid** (**TAT**), which was tested in rat models. The investigators concluded that TAT "possesses therapeutic value for the treatment of diabetic neuropathy."[59] It seems the Japanese never meet an ARI they do not like.)

My take on all of this is that although ARIs may be helpful in reducing sorbitol levels and thus ameliorating the symptoms of diabetic neuropathy, the penalty to be paid in terms of adverse events is too great to garner government approvals, at least in the U.S.

3. Ziconotide

This drug is a **synthetic analogue** (i.e., a structurally similar chemical) of a **peptide** isolated from the venom of ocean snails. Known as *conus magnus,* these little critters sting their prey with a lethal cocktail of neurotoxins injected through a harpoon-like tube. The venom from the *conus magus* is potent enough to paralyze a fish in a few seconds.

As manufactured into **ziconotide,** the peptide is a voltage-sensitive, N-type neuronal calcium "**channel**

---

[59] *Diabetes Research and Clinical Practice* (2001 Jan 1; 51(1): 9–20).

blocker." In effect it blocks the passage of pain-signaling calcium ions at channel entryways into nerve cells.

Some reports claim ziconotide is as much as **1000** times more effective than morphine as a pain-killer.

In February 2000, Elan Corporation, the manufacturer of ziconotide, announced that its New Drug Application had been accepted as filed by the FDA. The company said that positive results from an unpublished Phase III clinical trial of the drug's use in more than 700 patients with intractable pain led to the acceptance. Reportedly, significant pain relief was achieved in 57% of patients with neuropathic pain who had not attained relief with systemic opioid therapy. On June 28, 2000, the FDA issued an "approvable letter."[60] As of the time this was written the company had not received a final marketing go-ahead. (I spoke with an Elan representative in February 2001. She said the company was still going "through a few hoops" for the FDA. She did not want to speculate as to when final approval for the product could be expected.)

In October 2000, DRAXIS Health, Inc., the Canadian licensee of ziconotide, said it had filed a New Drug Submission with the Therapeutic Products Programme of Health Canada on a Priority Review basis. (The CEO of DRAXIS noted that in 1999 only eight of 84 NDS submissions were selected for Priority Review, an indication in his opinion of the drug's potential importance.)

---

[60] FDA issues "approvable letters" to manufacturers when remaining questions need to be resolved before final marketing approval can be granted.

Ziconotide definitely looks like one of the brighter stars in the galaxy of hopefuls for the treatment of neuropathic pain.

4. Zonisamide

Zonisamide is an anticonvulsant drug which is said to exert its effects through **sodium** and **calcium channel blockade** as well as through **dopaminergic** (relating to the neurotransmitter dopamine) and **serotonergic** (relating to the neurotransmitter serotonin) activity.

Investigators at the University of Wisconsin Hospitals in Madison, Wisconsin, recently conducted a study to determine appropriate dose ranges and evaluate the safety of the drug in humans with neuropathic pain.[61] (Zonisamide had previously been found effective in relieving neuropathic pain in animal models.) Thirteen patients were given doses starting at 25 mg daily or every other day, according to patient weights, and were increased weekly until the eighth week or until maximum tolerated dosage was reached. (The drug was said to be well tolerated up to doses of 300 mg.) Adverse events were generally considered mild. Further results were not available when this was written.

Larger studies to determine the efficacy, analgesic dose-range and safety of Zonisamide for treating neuropathic pain are said to be under way.

---

[61] Program and Abstracts of the 19th Annual Scientific Meeting of the American Pain Society; November 2–5, 2000; Atlanta, Georgia. Abstract 681.

Chapter 7

Some Other Matters

Since writing *Toes and Soles* I have kept a file of information—some of it perhaps a little "off the wall"—which you might find interesting or amusing or, in some cases, possibly useful.

Two Unusual Neuropathies

In an investigation of "**handcuff neuropathies,**" two clinicians conducted a 27-month prospective study at a large teaching hospital of all patients with a complaint of hand numbness, weakness, or *paresthesia*s attributed to overtightened handcuffs.[1] In the study, electrodiagnostic testing was performed on 18 subjects, and 41 were examined clinically. In the former group, neuropathies caused by the handcuffs were found in 22 superficial radial nerves, 12 were found in median nerves, and 9 were found in ulnar nerves. The clinicians found that the injuries to the latter two kinds of nerves were generally mild but that the handcuff-related injury to the most commonly af-

[1] *Muscle and Nerve* (2000 Jun; 23(6): 933–38).

fected nerve, the superficial radial, "can be severe and permanent." ("Loosen up there a little, man, you numbing my trigger finger.")

Another interesting study was labeled, "Heavy Snorer's Disease: A Progressive Local Neuropathy."[2] The investigators noted that chronic vibration of a tissue may cause neuronal damage leading to neuropathies. Referring to various studies, they said that a majority of patients with heavy snoring and different degrees of respiratory disturbance had signs of **pharyngeal** (i.e., relating to the pharynx) **nerve lesions** which could cause collapse of the upper airways. ("Turn over, Harry. We're out of Neurontin.")

Novel Causes

We always hear that there are "over 100 different causes of peripheral neuropathy." (One commentator says it is more like 200.) *Toes and Soles* listed a number of the more common ones, including diabetes, certain toxins and poisons, excessive alcohol intake, nutritional deficiencies and imbalances, and various diseases and disorders. Following are a few out-of-the-ordinary ones:

1. Statin Drugs

It may alarm some people to learn that **statin drugs,** commonly prescribed for coronary artery disease, can

---

[2] *Acta Oto-Laryngologica* (1999; 119(8): 925–33).

cause peripheral neuropathy.[3] Investigators reported a case of a patient who had been on **lipid-lowering** drug therapy with **lovastatin** after dietary therapy failed to lower his LDL cholesterol.[4] After four and a half years he began to complain of burning sensations in both feet and after several more months, gait disability. Neurological examinations and nerve conduction studies indicated PN. When the lovastatin was withdrawn his neuropathy improved significantly but never completely vanished.

Other lipid-lowering agents were administered over the next three years when the patient's LDL levels began to increase again but PN symptoms returned with each statin drug tried. Eventually that therapy was discontinued altogether. During the course of these other administrations, **niacin** (**vitamin B3**) was also used but the clinicians found that it exacerbated the patient's symptoms.[5]

---

[3] Statin drugs have been one of the most successful classes of drugs ever developed. Since the first statin, Mevacor (lovastatin), was released in 1988, randomized double-blind clinical trials have demonstrated significant mortality benefit and reductions in adverse events—myocardial infarction, bypass surgery, angioplasty and stroke.

[4] *Southern Medical Journal* (1998 Jul; 91(7): 667–68).

[5] *Toes and Soles* indicated that niacin, often used to reduce high cholesterol, usually helps in the proper functioning of the nervous system and in particular has been found helpful in rebuilding myelin sheath. I wonder if the result with niacin in the study reported here would indicate either a harmful synergistic effect when used with statin drugs, or could it mean that any method adopted to lower LDL cholesterol carries a risk of intensifying PN symptoms? (The researchers in the above study advised practitioners to consider all cholesterol-reducing agents as potential problems.) That would seem to run counter to the known fact that high LDL cholesterol levels

The investigators reviewed 45 cases of peripheral neuropathy associated with drugs such as lovastatin, simvastatin, and pravastatin. They said they found that once a statin produces a neuropathy, then "rechallenging with any of the other statins would likely cause a recurrence of the symptoms." They added that "the majority of cases appear to become manifested between 6 months and 2 years after therapy is started."

Another study reported seven cases of peripheral neuropathy caused by statins.[6] The investigators found that neuropathic symptoms persisted for ten weeks to a year in four cases after the statin treatment had been withdrawn.

2. Glue-sniffing Intoxication

This was a case report of a 24 year old female who had been sniffing glue and whose symptoms began with a progressive weakness in the lower extremities.[7] Neurological examination showed a decreased Achilles reflex response. The disorder continued to worsen for two weeks after the cessation of intoxication, with persistent evidence of "ongoing demyelination." Improvement was not observed for 40 days.

---

increase the danger, for example, of incurring diabetic neuropathy. (See, e.g., *Diabetes Research and Clinical Practice,* 2000 Nov 1; 50 Suppl 3:S15-S46). An interesting area for more research I would think.

[6] *European Journal of Clinical Pharmacology* (1999 Jan; 54(11): 835–38).

[7] *Tunisie Medicale* (1999 Nov; 77(11): 597–600).

3. *Mothball Abuse*

The authors of this study noted that **inhalant abuse** is a major public health problem associated with numerous acute and chronic medical problems; they said, though, that mothball abuse itself was "rare."[8] In this case the patient who had inhaled mothball fumes (hard to imagine anyone wanting to do that!) had "acute peripheral neuropathy and chronic renal failure." The clinicians reviewed the medical complications of the chemicals used in mothballs—napthalene and a certain type of benzene. They made the point that the misuse of common household products not usually identified as recreational drugs can cause serious problems such as peripheral neuropathy.

4. *Herpes*

Two clinicians presented a case in Spain of a 33 year old woman who developed "acute sensory neuropathy" after being diagnosed with an acute **varicella-zoster,** or **herpes,** virus infection which can cause chicken pox. All other causes of neuropathy had been ruled out, leaving the virus infection as the only possible explanation.[9]

---

[8] *Southern Medical Journal* (2000 Apr; 93(4): 427–29).

[9] *Revista de Neurologia* (1999 Jun 1–15; 28(11): 1067–69). There are ironical twists here and in the immediately preceding section concerning niacin-associated peripheral neuropathy. In each case the offending agent—niacin or the herpes virus—was deemed to have contributed to (niacin) or caused (herpes virus) the neuropathy. Yet in each case the active agent also is used in alleviating PN. (As discussed previously, studies of animal models have shown that a

5. Sports-related Injuries

These generally result in **entrapment** or **compression** neuropathies involving the **ulnar, suprascapular, peroneal** or **obturator** nerves. Four recent studies were found, relating to baseball, volley ball, surfing and soccer/ football injuries.

A study of neurological injuries in **baseball** players noted that injuries to the throwing arm of pitchers are quite common due to the extreme stresses placed on the elbow and shoulder joints.[10] These result in such peripheral nerve disorders as **ulnar neuropathy** at the elbow and **suprascapular neuropathy** at the shoulder. The researchers warn that repeated trauma causing aneurysms and thrombus formations could possibly lead to stroke.

Prolonged **wave-surfing** was found to have produced a **peroneal neuropathy** in one case.[11] The investigators in that study noted that this type of neuropathy among children and adolescents is usually caused by direct injury at the **fibular head** level.

Although **suprascapular nerve entrapment** is not common, it has been reported in **volleyball** players. In a recent study, 16 professional players of a Belgium male volleyball team underwent shoulder testing.[12] Four were found to have "severe suprascapular neuropathy."

---

modified herpes virus can carry nerve growth factor to damaged nerve sites.)

[10] *Seminars in Neurology* (2000; 20(2): 187–93).

[11] *Journal of Child Neurology* (2000 Jun; 15(6): 420–21).

[12] *British Journal of Sports Medicine* (2000 Jun; 34(3): 174–80).

In each the entrapment was on the **dominant side.** Significant differences between the affected and non-affected players were found for all shoulder range-of-motion measurements.

Entrapment neuropathies involving the **obturator nerve** are usually the result of vigorous exercise in such games as **soccer** and **football.**[13] Patients who have this condition typically complain of an insidious onset of **groin pain,** which they describe as a deep ache centered on the adductor origin at the pubic bone. During exercise the pain is more severe and may radiate down the medial aspect of the thigh toward the knee. They may also notice exercise-related weakness in the affected leg when they attempt to jump. Patients seldom report numbness or *paresthesia,* except in cases lasting longer than 12 months.

6. "Telesales" Neuropathy

A case was reported at the Department of Neurology, St. James's University Hospital, in Leeds, England, of a **bilateral ulnar neuropathy** caused by **overuse** of a **telephone.**[14] The patient was described as a 17-year old "double glazing salesman" making sales calls. (We have had a few 17-year olds in our family who, I'll venture, used the phone every bit as much as the boy in England. I don't

[13] *The Physician and Sportsmedicine* (1999 May; 27(5)).
[14] *Postgrad Med J* (2000 Dec; 76(902): 793–94).

think, though, that their purpose was ever as worthwhile as his.)

7. A "Shocking" Cause

The British medical journal, *The Lancet,* recently reported on what had appeared to be an unfathomable case of diabetic neuropathy.[15] It seems that a man came to a diabetes clinic complaining of excessive thirst and excessive urination, blurred vision, and appreciable, sudden weight loss. He had no other symptoms and there was no evidence at the time of sensory neuropathy. He was treated with insulin and given a prescription for another medication. The patient returned to the clinic three months later for a routine follow-up, accompanied by his wife. He felt well, he said, in general, and had resumed work as a carpenter. His only complaint was of *paresthesia* in his hands and feet that he described as "kind of like an electric shock." He worried that these symptoms might be an early sign of diabetic nerve damage. His physician, perhaps thinking he had somehow missed not having diagnosed a neuropathy earlier and realizing the patient was describing a classic sign of peripheral neuropathy when he mentioned electric shocks, proceeded to outline the benefits of strict glucose control.

After listening intently for several minutes the patient seemed convinced. "I didn't know whether or not I should be worried," he said. "After all, I only get the tingling

[15] *The Lancet* (2000 Apr 29; 355 (9214): 1560).

when I'm taking a shower. When I reach up and adjust the shower head, I feel it in my hand—and it feels like its coming out my feet."

"You know, I've felt the same thing," his non-diabetic wife suddenly volunteered. The patient and his wife were immediately referred to a specialist in that kind of syndrome—an electrician—who found that the grounding of the electrical system in their house was dangerously faulty. The defect was promptly repaired and their symptoms completely resolved. The author of the *Lancet* article reminded that things are not always as they seem.

8. Both a Cure and a Cause

The NMDA receptor antagonist **amantadine** (a class of drugs which includes memantine, discussed previously), has been demonstrated to be effective in treating neuropathic pain. Three patients had their symptoms completely resolved by the administration of this compound in one study.[16]

However in another study a 48-year old woman developed a "peripheral sensory-motor neuropathy" because of the eight-year administration of amantadine. Discontinuation of the drug resulted in a complete resolution of her symptoms, according to the investigators.[17]

---

[16] *Pain* (1998 Feb; 74(2–3): 337–39). However in another study, lidocaine was found superior to amantadine for sciatica, a neuropathic pain syndrome caused by compression and/or inflammation of spinal nerve roots. *Regional Anesthesia and Pain Medicine* (1999 Nov-Dec; 24(6): 534–40).

[17] *Neurology* (1999 Nov 10; 53(8): 1862–65).

Other Drug Causes

Following is a list of other drugs said to cause peripheral neuropathy, compiled from various sources. Incidentally, you will note a few (e.g., Elavil, Dilantin) often prescribed to *treat* PN, just as with the example above:

alfa interferon (Roferon-A, Intron A, Alferon N)
amiodarone (Cordarone)
amitriptyline (Elavil)
chloroquine (Aralen)
cimetidine (Tagamet)
cisplatin (Platinol)
colchicine (Probenecid)
ddC (Hivid)
ddI (Videx)
d4T (Stavudine)
dapsone
dioxin
disulfiram (Antabuse)
dolostatin-10
ethambutol (Myambutol)
FIAU
hydralazine (Apresoline)
isoniazid (Laniazid)
lithium phenytoin (Dilantin)
lovastatin (Mevacor)
metronidazole (Flagyl)
nitrous oxide
paclitaxel (Taxol)
pravastatin (Pravachol)
pyridoxine (Nestrex, Beesix)
simvastatin (Zocor)
stavudine (Zerit)

suramin (Fourneau 309, Bayer 205, Germanin)
thalidomide (Synovir)
vincristine (Oncovin)
zalcitabine[18]

Prevalence of Idiopathic Neuropathies

Generally it is assumed that about one third of neuropathies are from unknown causes and are therefore "**idiopathic.**" A study in Vienna, Austria, retrospectively examined the efficacy of standard procedures used in the diagnosis of peripheral neuropathy. Both non-invasive and invasive measures were considered. In an in-depth analysis of 171 patients, non-invasive investigations were sufficient to reveal the underlying PN cause in 81% of patients. In the other 19% the cause remained idiopathic.[19] The investigators indicated that if **invasive** measures such as **nerve** or **skin biopsies** had been employed, even fewer of those neuropathies would have been classified idiopathic. The idea here is that with a little further "poking around," the mysteries behind idiopathic neuropathies can often be unraveled.

---

[18] This antiretroviral has sometimes been used in the long-term management of HIV infections. Its use has been restricted, though, because of its perceived potential for inducing PN. Recent studies have shown, however, that peripheral neuropathy is relatively infrequent when zalcitabine is used in combination with other antiretrovirals. *International Journal of STD and AIDS* (2000 Jul; 11(7): 417–23).

[19] *Postgraduate Medical Journal* (1999 Dec; 75(890): 723–27).

More HIV/AIDS Neuropathies Coming

Peripheral neuropathy is thought to be the most common pain syndrome experienced by people with HIV infections. (It is also the most common complication in people with diabetes.) Because **highly active anti-retroviral therapy** (**HAART**) is increasingly available which itself can cause PN,[20] experts think it unlikely that its incidence will decrease among the HIV/AIDS population. Dr. David Clifford, a neuropathy specialist in St. Louis, has been quoted as saying he thinks the neuropathy rate could be as high as 50% or more in PWAs already because of the high-powered **combination therapies** being used capable of causing neurological problems. (The range that generally has been accepted is 30 to 35%.) Justin McArthur, M.D., a neurologist at Johns Hopkins seconds this observation, saying, "We will see a lot more toxic neuropathy with long-term use of these combinations."

There is another aspect to the increasing use of HAART which almost surely will produce even more cases of HIV-related neuropathy. According to a news story from *Reuters* which appeared just as this was writ-

[20] "Nucleoside analogue reverse transcriptase inhibitors represent an important contributor to peripheral neuropathy. Specifically, around 10% of patients receiving stavudine or zalcitabine and 1 to 2% of didanosine recipients may have to discontinue therapy with these agents due to neuropathy." *Drug Safety* (1998 Dec; 19(6): 481–94).

ten, a "rebound epidemic" of HIV was occurring in San Francisco and other urban centers where relatively high populations of gay young men are living. One of the reasons given was the emergence of "successful new AIDS drug treatments." According to the story, the advent of these treatments was causing the gay community to drop its guard, with many members engaging in riskier behavior, leading to more cases of HIV infections, resulting in still more cases of peripheral neuropathy, leading to more combination therapies, causing . . . . Get the picture? It is a sad one of a vicious trend feeding on itself.

An Early Description of Neuropathic Pain

A physician by the name of S. Weir Mitchell described neuropathic pain in his 1872 book, *Injuries of Nerves and Their Consequences,* and documented a number of cases in Civil war patients.

He wrote that the area directly affected in these men typically became "exquisitely hyperaesthetic, so that a touch or a tap of the finger increases the pain."

Patients took great lengths to avoid exposing the area to the air, he reported. "Most of the bad cases keep the hand constantly wet, finding relief in the moisture rather than in the coolness of the application."

And he could see that this kind of pain took a heavy toll. "As the pain increases, the general sympathy becomes more marked. The temper changes and grows irritable, the face becomes anxious, and has a look of weariness and suffering. The sleep is restless, and the constitutional condition. . . . exasperates the hyperaesthetic state, so that the rattling of a newspaper, a breath of air . . . the vibrations caused by a military band, or the shock of the feet in walking, gives rise to increase of pain."

Any of this sound familiar?

Finding a Doctor

A question many PNers ask is, "Where can I find a good doctor in my area?" The answer is not always easy to come by, and there are few places to turn for objective information.

One suggestion sometimes mentioned is state or local medical directories. In my opinion, though, you might as well go to the yellow pages in your telephone directory for all the help you will generally get there. Besides specialty and contact information, the only relevant fact usually mentioned is whether the doctor has faced disciplinary actions.

Of course, members of the Neuropathy Association looking for a neurologist have access to a list of "Neuropathy Clinical Centers" across the country at the web site, *www.neuropathy.org*. A number of these doctors are associated with major teaching institutions in large cities.

However, they may be inaccessible to many PNers both for geographical reasons and because they often have extremely busy schedules. (I guess it would raise a red flag if they were not!)

If you are able to get opinions of other PNers on the subject (one of the benefits of belonging to a local neuropathy support group is that you can exchange such information), you may come up with names of neurologists or other doctors who have been found to be helpful to your new friends.

In an article in the *American Journal of Public Health* (November 4, 1997), on finding "good doctors," the authors reported on surveys based on **patient outcomes.** Their conclusion was that **experience** in a particular discipline counts more than anything in picking a doctor. They noted, for example, that the patient mortality ratio following bypass surgeries was lowest for physicians who performed more than 400 in a three-year period. That is well and good—and maybe slightly obvious—but how are you really going to be able to find out, for example, which neurologists in your area deal with the most cases of peripheral neuropathy (and if the hypothesis holds, which have therefore been most successful in treating their patients' neuropathy complaints)? I don't think there is any good way we can determine these things without spending a lot of time and irritating a lot of doctors' secretaries with what they may perceive as none-of-your-business questions.

There is help out there, though! A friend gave me an interesting book entitled, *Guide to Top Doctors,* which I do think offers practical assistance in finding a medical practitioner, whether it be a neurologist or another specialist.

The book is a listing of the 15,000 "top-rated physicians" in America's largest metropolitan areas, with ratings based on the number of *recommendations from other doctors.*

The idea is that since doctors who are looking for medical help for themselves often ask other doctors for recommendations, a **compilation** of these **recommendations** could help others make good choices. (The concept makes sense to me. I have often asked doctors for their recommendations in fields in which they don't practice; it's a "word gets around" idea. Of course if you ask them for recommendations in their own practice field, they may not take too kindly to your question!)

Doctors are listed in that book both by geographical area and medical specialty. Every listing provides background information on the doctor—including medical school attended and any "board certifications"—and indicates how many times the particular doctor was recommended by other doctors in his or her geographical area.

The recommendations were taken from a survey of about 260,000 physicians in more than 50 of the largest Metropolitan Statistical areas in the U.S. who were on the mailing list of the American Medical Association. This should be a large enough universe that biases ("she goes to my church") and favoritism ("you recommend me, partner, and I will recommend you") should be substantially reduced.

More information on the book can be found at *www.checkbook*.org.

Working with Your Doctor

There was an interesting article in the March 1999 issue of the *Ladies' Home Journal* (my thanks to a lady who brought it to my attention) on how to get the most out of the doctor/patient relationship—from the patient's point of view. Following are some of the suggestions given:

- Educate yourself (just as you are doing now). Your doctor should not be your only source of information. For example, pharmacists and patient support groups (such as member groups of the Neuropathy Association) can provide useful information.
- If you have an article from a newspaper or magazine, or a book (*Toes and Soles*? This book?), you would like to discuss with your doctor, don't be reluctant to take the material with you to your appointment.
- For your initial session, bring in all your medications—prescription as well as over-the-counter. Also be prepared to discuss your symptoms in detail.
- Be willing as well to discuss your medical history in depth. Don't be afraid to divulge information that might be relevant. Your doctor will be much more effective in dealing with your problem if he or she knows as much about the surrounding circumstances as you do.
- Be honest. Even if it's uncomfortable admitting to unhealthy behavior, it is necessary to tell your doc-

tor the truth. (You need to admit "I prefer a tumbler of bourbon to a glass of orange juice as soon as I wake up," if such is the case.)

- Take notes and if the explanation is complex, have your doctor write it down for you.
- If you disagree with what your doctor is prescribing, do it in a way not to put him or her on the defensive. Perhaps say something such as, "May I have your thinking on this?" (You'll get a much better reaction than asking, "How many of your patients have died from stupid advice like that?")
- Get a second opinion if your doctor advises an invasive test or therapy that carries risk. According to C. Edward Rose, M.D., professor of medicine at the University of Virginia School of Medicine, "Any physician who has the interest of the patient in mind should welcome a second opinion to ensure he's giving the right recommendation."[21]

An article in *The Journal of the American Medical Association,* "How to Talk with Your Doctor," made many of the same points, emphasizing that you need to be as specific as possible in describing your symptoms and health concerns, including when the symptoms started, what they feel like, any lifestyle changes you made when

[21] *Toes and Soles* underscored the fact that *you* are the final arbiter of your own situation. If your doctor isn't meeting your needs, express your concerns. If he or she still "doesn't get it," find another doctor.

they started, anything in particular that triggers them, or anything that relieves your symptoms.[22]

Looking at the doctor/patient relationship from the opposite point of view, the same issue of *JAMA* reported an interesting study of 1057 audiotaped encounters between doctors and their patients.[23] The investigators found that in nine out of ten decisions made between doctors and patients in routine office visits, the *doctors* failed to discuss the patient's problem sufficiently to allow the *patient* to make an informed choice. Something important was missing 91% of the time, such as talking about the pros and cons, and various implications of a decision. One example was doctors failing to note that there could be unpleasant side effects when indicating that a higher dose of a particular medication might offer more relief.

In an editorial on that study, still in the same issue, Michael J. Barry, M.D., Massachusetts General Hospital, Boston, had the following observation on the problem of doctors' paternalism, as he put it:

> Why do physicians appear to be so paternalistic in day-to-day office practice? Physicians most likely would argue that there is simply insufficient time to adopt the shared decision-making approach, particularly in the current managed care era, in which most office-based physicians feel pressured to see an increasing number of patients in the same amount of time. In fact, the encounters with primary care physicians in this study averaged about 16 minutes in duration, and a median of

---

[22] *JAMA* (1999 Dec 22/29; 282(24): 2422).
[23] Ibid., (2313–20).

> 3 patient concerns were tackled. In such a visit, basic history taking and a focused physical examination will usually precede a discussion about diagnostic and therapeutic options; physicians may simply tell patients what to do without much elaboration to move on to the next examination room quickly.

As far as solving the problem is concerned, Dr. Barry had the following to offer:

> Trying to explain, in a balanced way, the complex issues behind controversies such as whether to perform a PSA test or prescribe estrogen replacement therapy cannot be done quickly. For decisions that must be faced routinely in office practice, educational materials such as pamphlets, videotapes, or even interactive videodiscs may be helpful for communicating basic information about a decision and the possible outcomes of different management options, so that clinicians' limited time can be spent not on basic education, but on tailoring the management strategy to the patient's preferences.

I hope your doctor is sincerely interested in trying to fully communicate with you but remember, it's a two-way street.

Patient Assistance

Toes and Soles discussed patience assistance programs, whereby major drug companies *give* their products to people who cannot afford to buy them. These programs, which are particularly appealing to seniors, appear to be proliferating. In 1999 a total of 2.7 million prescriptions valued at about $500 million were provided without charge to people who met the criteria set by pharmaceutical companies.

It is not just "poor people" who qualify. Often, approved candidates are those who earn too much to get government assistance but are pinched because they have high medical costs and do not have insurance to pay for prescriptions. Patient-advocacy groups indicate, in fact, that families earning $50,000 or even more have qualified under these programs.

Not all drugs are included in these give-aways but a number of well-known medications are. A listing of drugs and drug manufacturers involved in various programs is set out at the web site *www.cancercareinc.org/services/drug_companies.htm.* (Don't be put off by the reference to cancer in the web address—drugs such as Neurontin and Tegretol in which we are interested are included.) Also there is a very complete list of various drug companies with patient assistance programs at the web site, *www.phrma.org.* Click on the links to the various companies listed there and you can determine which drugs they include in their programs, as well as program criteria and procedures.

One site that I think would be particularly useful is *www.needymeds.com.* As of the time this was written 966 drugs available in patient assistance programs were listed. The best thing about the information there is that all of the drugs are alphabetically listed, with hotlinks directly to the company's site for each drug. This eliminates the need to know in advance which pharmaceutical company manufactures which drug you wish to check. Included are old favorites such as clonidine, Dilantin, EMLA cream, Klonopin, Lamictal, and Neurontin.

Talking about patient-help web sites, there is one which provides a variety of services to those seeking a means to travel long-distances for specialized medical evaluation, diagnosis and treatment but who cannot afford to pay for their own travel. Called the National Patient Travel Helpline, information is provided concerning various forms of charitable medical air transportation as well as referrals to appropriate sources of help through the Angel Flight America Network. The Helpline can reached at 1-800-296-1217and is available 24 hours a day, seven days a week.

There is also an organization which provides free lodging and support services to families of limited means who are away from their home while one of their members is receiving medical treatment. Called the National Association of Hospital Hospitality Houses, Inc., the organization operates through a national network of "hospitality member/houses." Information concerning their services may be obtained by calling 1-800-542-9730.

Where to Find More on Disability Coping

If you wanted to go to just one site to find information on disabilities, you probably could do no better than visiting *http://www.disabilityresources.org.* They cover about everything on the subject you could think of. Also the people who run it publish an excellent newsletter called, *Disability Resources Monthly.* Each issue is chock full of ideas to "help people with disabilities live, learn, love, work and play independently," as they say in their mission statement. Recent issues, for example, contained features on new technologies such as home automation equipment (voice controlled telephones, remote controlled lighting, etc.); a reference to a video—Senior Solutions—concerning some low-tech ways of coping for those with physical or cognitive problems; and a number of reviews of books written on such subjects as basic advice to parents of children with disabilities. The newsletter can be ordered by calling 631-585-0290.

The Muscular Dystrophy Association publishes a paper entitled "101 Hints to 'Help-with-Ease' for Patients with Neuromuscular Disease: A Do-It-Yourself Owner's Guide," which also has many suggestions for *anyone* suffering a disability. All the "hints" it contains have been field-tested and proven useful, according to the authors, one who is an M.D. and directs M.D.A clinics, the other an occupational therapist. The hints are designed to help patients and their caregivers tend to daily tasks of "eating, grooming, dressing, sitting, transferring, communicating, getting around, using the toilet, working, recreating, traveling, shopping and sleeping," which doesn't leave out much. The article can be accessed on line at *http://www.M.D.ausa.org/publications/101hints/index.html.* While there I suggest you click on "additional devices" at the bottom of the opening page. That will take you to a page offering contact information for companies with free catalogs describing devices and aids for the disabled.

Another excellent site concerning "personal care" products can be found at *http://www.abledata.com.* Check out *http://4disability.4anything.com/4/0,1001,3096,00.html,* as well on the same subject.

There is also an association which has a good deal of information at their web site, the American Association of People with Disabilities. Go to *http://www.aapd.com/info/* and then click on "Other Sites" for a list of additional resources.

Another web site, this one across the pond from us, with even more links to various other Internet URLs, is *http://www.soon.org.uk/problems/disability.htm.* Not only can you click through to various organizational resources but also to indices listing newsletters, newsgroups, forums, bulletin boards and chat rooms which may be of interest to PNers who don't function as well as they used to. (Ain't the Internet just grand?)

Last but (hopefully) not least, there is a recommended reading list at *www.medpress.com* which has information on several books concerning coping with pain and disabilities (as well as a number of other subjects covered in this book).

Thank you for reading my book. I hope it has given you some ideas that will help you.

If you are interested in further information concerning peripheral neuropathy, particularly nutrient supplementation, or relieving neuropathy pain, please send your request to MedPress, Box 81 Halifax, Nova Scotia, Canada, B3J 2L4.

Thank you.

John Senneff
July 2001

BOOK ORDER FORM

Order extra copies for any friends or relatives you think might benefit – even for your doctor!)

Telephone orders: Call 1-888-MED-9898 toll free (1-888-633-9898)

Fax orders: Fax the form you have filled in below to 1-902-492-0013

Postal orders: Mail the form you have filled in below to:

MedPress, PO Box 81 Halifax,
Nova Scotia, Canada B3J 2L4

Please send me the following:

Nutrients for Neuropathy

_____ copies (paperback), $19.95 each

Numb Toes and Aching Soles: Coping with Peripheral Neuropathy

_____ copies (paperback), $24.95 each

_____ copies (professional case bound edition), $31.95 each

Numb Toes and Other Woes: More on Peripheral Neuropathy

_____ copies (paperback), $24.95 each

_____ copies (professional case bound edition), $31.95 each

Shipping & Handling

Please add for U.S. deliveries, $7 for first book, $3 for each additional book. For shipments outside the U.S., please call 1-888-234-7256 or email HYPERLINK "mailto:orders@medpress.com" orders@ medpress.com for information.

Payment: _____ Check (payable to "MedPress")

_____ Credit Card:
The undersigned hereby consents to payment for orders to be charged to a credit card listed below:

Authorised Signature: ______________________________

Print Name on Card: ______________________________ Date: ________

Credit Card Number: ______________________________

Card Type: ____________________ (Visa, Mastercard or AMEX)

Exp Date: __________

3-Digit Code (req'd): _______

Corresponding Address for Credit Card: ______________________________

____

Corresponding Telephone Number
for Credit Card: ______________________________

Index